OTHER *ESSENTIALS* BOOKS

Essentials for the NEW NURSE PRACTITIONER: What You Really Need to Know in a Nutshell (*Aktan*)

Essentials for the A&E NURSE: Emergency Department Orientation in a Nutshell (*Buettner*)

Essentials About GI AND LIVER DISEASES FOR NURSES: What APRNs Need to Know in a Nutshell (*Chaney*)

Essentials on COMBATTING NURSE BULLYING, INCIVILITY, AND WORKPLACE VIOLENCE: What Nurses Need to Know in a Nutshell (*Ciocco*)

Essentials for the THEATRE NURSE: An Orientation and Care Guide in a Nutshell (*Criscitelli*)

Essentials for the NEONATAL NURSE: A Nursing Orientation and Care Guide in a Nutshell (*Davidson*)

Essentials for the LONG-TERM CARE NURSE: What Nursing Home and Assisted Living Nurses Need to Know in a Nutshell (*Eliopoulos*)

Essentials for the CLINICAL NURSE MANAGER: Managing a Changing Workplace in a Nutshell (*Fry*)

Essentials for EVIDENCE-BASED PRACTICE: Implementing EBP in a Nutshell (*Godshall*)

Essentials for Nurses About HOME INFUSION THERAPY: The Expert's Best Practice Guide in a Nutshell (*Gorski*)

Essentials for MIDWIVES: Labour & Delivery Orientation in a Nutshell (*Groll*)

Essentials for the RADIOLOGY NURSE: An Orientation and Nursing Care Guide in a Nutshell (*Grossman*)

Essentials for the CARDIAC SURGERY NURSE: Caring for Cardiac Surgery Patients in a Nutshell (*Hodge*)

Essentials for DEMENTIA CARE: What Nurses Need to Know in a Nutshell (*Miller*)

Essentials for STROKE CARE NURSING: An Expert Guide in a Nutshell (*Morrison*)

Essentials for the PAEDIATRIC NURSE: An Orientation Guide in a Nutshell (*Rupert, Young*)

Essentials for the TRIAGE NURSE: An Orientation and Care Guide in a Nutshell (*Visser, Montejano, Grossman*)

Essentials for the HOSPICE NURSE: A Concise Guide to End-of-Life Care (*Wright*)

Essentials About PTSD: A Guide for Nurses and Other Health Care Professionals (*Adams*)

Essentials for the CLINICAL NURSING INSTRUCTOR: Clinical Teaching in a Nutshell (*Kan, Stabler-Haas*)

Essentials for MANAGING PATIENTS WITH A PSYCHIATRIC DISORDER: What RNs, NPs, and New Psych Nurses Need to Know (*Marshall*)

Essentials About the GYNAECOLOGIC EXAM: A Professional Guide for NPs, PAs, and Midwives (*Secor, Fantasia*)

ESSENTIALS for the **CLINICAL NURSING INSTRUCTOR**

Eden Zabat Kan, PhD, RN, received her bachelor's degree in nursing from Penn State University, State College, Pennsylvania; her master's degree in nursing education from Villanova University, Villanova, Pennsylvania; and her doctorate in nursing science from Widener University, Chester, Pennsylvania. She is currently employed in the nursing department, Health Sciences Division, the College of Southern Maryland, La Plata, Maryland.

Susan Stabler-Haas, PMHCNS-BC, RN, is a clinical instructor at Villanova University, Villanova, Pennsylvania. She has more than 30 years of classroom and clinical teaching experience in the areas of medical–surgical, critical care, geriatric, and psychiatric nursing. Her instruction is influenced by her prior roles as staff nurse, rehabilitation nurse, and critical care nurse manager in five Philadelphia-area hospitals. Professor Stabler-Haas has earned a psychiatric clinical nurse specialist designation from the University of Pennsylvania. She is a licensed marriage and family therapist, a trained mindfulness-based meditation teacher, and author of *Essentials for the Student Nurse*.

ESSENTIALS for the CLINICAL NURSING INSTRUCTOR

Clinical Teaching in a Nutshell

Eden Zabat Kan, PhD, RN
Susan Stabler-Haas, PMHCNS-BC, RN

SPRINGER PUBLISHING COMPANY

Copyright © 2018 Springer Publishing Company, LLC

All rights reserved.

No part of this publication may be reproduced, stored in a retrieval system, or transmitted in any form or by any means, electronic, mechanical, photocopying, recording, or otherwise, without the prior permission of Springer Publishing Company, LLC, or authorization through payment of the appropriate fees to the Copyright Clearance Center, Inc., 222 Rosewood Drive, Danvers, MA 01923, 978-750-8400, fax 978-646-8600, info@copyright.com or on the Web at www.copyright.com.

Springer Publishing Company, LLC
11 West 42nd Street
New York, NY 10036
www.springerpub.com

Acquisitions Editor: Margaret Zuccarini
Senior Production Editor: Kris Parrish
Compositor: Westchester Publishing Services

ISBN: 978-0-8261-8817-5

17 18 19 20 / 5 4 3 2 1

The author and the publisher of this Work have made every effort to use sources believed to be reliable to provide information that is accurate and compatible with the standards generally accepted at the time of publication. Because medical science is continually advancing, our knowledge base continues to expand. Therefore, as new information becomes available, changes in procedures become necessary. We recommend that the reader always consult current research and specific institutional policies before performing any clinical procedure. The author and publisher shall not be liable for any special, consequential, or exemplary damages resulting, in whole or in part, from the readers' use of, or reliance on, the information contained in this book. The publisher has no responsibility for the persistence or accuracy of URLs for external or third-party Internet websites referred to in this publication and does not guarantee that any content on such websites is, or will remain, accurate or appropriate.

> Contact us to receive discount rates on bulk purchases.
> We can also customize our books to meet your needs.
> For more information please contact: sales@springerpub.com

The ESSENTIALS series was published in the United States by Springer Publishing Company, LLC, as the FAST FACTS series.

Contents

Preface xiii
Acknowledgments xvii
Introduction xix

Part I APPRECIATING YOUR NEW IDENTITY: FROM CAREGIVER TO EDUCATOR

1. Developing a New Identity as a Clinical Nursing Instructor   3
2. Understand the Rules: What Every Nursing Instructor Needs to Know About the Nursing Program's Policies   13
3. Your New World: Clinical Sites, Clinical Specialties, Clinical Students   23

Part II YOUR SUCCESS DEPENDS ON YOU: PREPARING FOR YOUR CLINICAL TEACHING ASSIGNMENT

4. You Are a Guest, So Act Like One   41
5. Organize the Semester—Have a Plan   47
6. Confidentiality and Patient Privacy   61

Part III GETTING TO KNOW YOUR NURSING STUDENTS: WHO ARE THE BEST AND WHO ARE THE REST?

7. The High Fliers: How to Screen for Higher Achieving Students — 69
8. The Not-So-High Fliers: How to Screen for Potential "Problem Students" — 73

Part IV THE PERFORMANCE APPRAISALS: CLINICAL EVALUATIONS

9. The Clinical Evaluation Triad — 83
10. The *Dos* and *Don'ts* of Student Documentation — 89
11. Early Warning System — 95
12. Graded Clinical Versus Pass/Fail Evaluations — 103

Part V MANAGING THE CLINICAL DAY

13. Preconferences — 111
14. Postconferences — 115
15. Unplanned Events and Absences — 121
16. Alternative Assignments — 127
17. Unsafe Practice — 135

Part VI SATISFACTION IN THE ROLE

18. What Your Students Will Expect of You — 143
19. Take Time for Self-Care — 153

Part VII OF GROWING IMPORTANCE

20. Letters of Reference — 163
21. Role of Simulation — 171

Appendices — *177*
   A. An Example of Guidelines for Clinical Orientation Day — *179*
   B. Clinical Journal: NSL/NSG 423 — *181*
   C. 4 C Clinical Assignment Sheet — *185*

    D. *Student Report Sheet*   *187*
    E. *One-Minute Breathing Space*   *197*
    F. *Sample Letters of Reference*   *199*
Bibliography   *203*
Index   *205*

Preface

The dream begins with a teacher who believes in you, who tugs and pushes and leads you to the next plateau, sometimes poking you with a sharp stick called "truth."
—Dan Rather

For those of you teaching nursing and those aspiring to teach nursing, has there ever been a time when Dan Rather's words resounded more loudly than they do today? Although compassion for others will always remain its essence, nursing continues to become more and more complex. Therein lies the challenge: ensuring that our students' hearts remain firmly invested in the patient as a person, while developing the agility of their minds to process a swift and steady stream of technical innovation in the discharge of their accountability. In order to teach our students well, we need to be willing to tug and push and lead all of them to the next plateau. On our journey, the sharp stick of truth is the most important of all tools that we must carry in our "clinical nursing instructor backpack"—truth in teaching both the ideals and the realities of nursing in today's health care environment.

Not every nurse makes a good clinical instructor. Technical proficiency alone does not guarantee the ability to effectively manage nursing students at the clinical site. Even nurses who are capable of providing clinical instruction may not wish to take on the considerable responsibility associated with the oversight of these nursing students.

Perhaps you are different. Perhaps you are a nurse who is both capable and willing to impart your knowledge to the next generation of caregivers. We commend you, for the future of our profession rests on your shoulders. After all, what is more important to the future of nursing than supervising and sharing our expertise with those who will follow us?

Although personally rewarding, this vital role is also a formidable challenge. Clinical teaching is not easy. The expectations for an effective clinical nursing instructor are daunting. It can be a prodigious undertaking even for individuals with training or degrees in clinical instruction. These instructors are continually faced with the changing demands of patients and the challenges of adapting instruction to different learning styles and the rapidly changing face of today's student nurses. As clinical instructors ourselves, we would like to share our own experiences in this regard in the hope that you will profit from them.

Is it important as a new clinical instructor to have a solid foundation in teaching clinical courses? Not necessarily. Indeed, many may not have any teaching experience. As a result, they face performance insecurities, along with the daily teaching challenges. It is easy to understand why nursing programs are pressed to fill clinical instructor positions. Couple this with the fact that the American Association of Colleges of Nursing (AACN) found that U.S. nursing schools turned away nearly 69,000 qualified applicants in 2014, partly because of a shortage of faculty, and you have the making of a crisis, according to Marcia Faller, PhD, RN, chief clinical officer at AMN Healthcare (as cited in Dishman, 2015).

Meanwhile, the American Nurses Association (ANA) is currently lobbying Congress to increase funding for Title VIII of the Public Health Service Act. The provision allots federal grants for nursing schools and organizations, so that they can advance their educational programs, promote diversity in the field, repay loans for nursing students who work in facilities with critical shortages, train geriatric nurses, and more (Grant, 2016).

Essentials for the Clinical Nursing Instructor: Clinical Teaching in a Nutshell is designed as a practical guide for current and aspiring clinical instructors. This book addresses key fundamental elements of clinical teaching. These elements include, but are not limited to, developing an identity as a new instructor; preparing for teaching; developing a student clinical assignment; conducting the student evaluation; and perhaps, most importantly, taking time for self-care (see Chapter 19). There is rich and valuable material throughout the book, such as exhibits with student examples, case scenarios, and case studies, which serve as resources and added support for the clinical instructor. Every chapter has been reviewed and updated to reflect the most recent changes in clinical education.

In short, we hope that this book will offer useful insights as you guide your students from one plateau of knowledge to the next. We wish you great success on that journey.

Eden Zabat Kan
Susan Stabler-Haas

References

Dishman, L. (2015). These will be the most in-demand jobs in 2016. Retrieved from https://www.fastcompany.com/3054142/the-future-of-work/these-will-be-the-most-in-demand-jobs-in-2016

Grant, R. (2016, February 3). The U.S. is running out of nurses. *The Atlantic*. Retrieved from https://www.theatlantic.com/health/archive/2016/02/nursing-shortage/459741/

Rather, D. (n.d.). Retrieved from https://www.brainyquote.com/quotes/quotes/d/danrather108025.html

Acknowledgments

To Alex and Christine for being wonderful and supportive when I write and work away from you. I am blessed to have found a career that I love with students and colleagues who are most supportive. Special thanks to my coauthor and friend, Sue; we have known each other for many years, but I still do miss our coffee chats after our clinical days at the hospital.

Eden Zabat Kan

I wish to thank all of my students whose feedback over the years has helped to shape this book. I also would like to thank my husband, Joe, for his support. Special thanks to all of my colleagues who shared their clinical-specialty expertise that appears in this book. To my coauthor, Eden; no one could ask for a better writing partner. Lastly, I would like to remember my dear friend Irene, a nurse who exemplified the true qualities of a human being. I will miss her.

Susan Stabler-Haas

Introduction

The major purpose of this book is to provide specific and practical information and guidelines for clinical nursing professors/instructors (these terms can be used interchangeably). Many of these professionals work exceedingly hard to perform a role, the complexities and frustrations of which are often underrecognized. A clinical nursing professor/instructor has one of the most challenging and potentially rewarding positions in the nursing profession. Today more than ever, it is a role that every state needs to fill in a multitude of programs.

> America's 3 million nurses make up the largest segment of the health-care workforce in the U.S., and nursing is currently one of the fastest-growing occupations in the country. Despite that growth, demand is outpacing supply. According to the Bureau of Labor Statistics, 1.2 million vacancies will emerge for registered nurses between 2014 and 2022. By 2025, the shortfall is expected to be "more than twice as large as any nurse shortage experienced since the introduction of Medicare and Medicaid in the mid-1960s," a team of Vanderbilt University nursing researchers wrote in a 2009 paper on the issue. (Grant, 2016, para. 4)

As the demand for new nurses continues to grow, this book should continue to be a valuable resource for those dedicated to the task of educating tomorrow's nursing professionals.

PURPOSE AND ORGANIZATION OF THIS BOOK

This book has seven major parts containing 21 chapters. The chapters provide elemental information applicable to all clinical professors/instructors. Some offer knowledge about the mechanics of clinical instruction, whereas others assist a new instructor in organizing his or her work. Within each chapter are exhibits that include sample templates or case scenarios and cases studies. We believe the exhibits and case studies incorporated into the chapters provide rich insight that can further support clinical instruction. However, this book does not provide all the information necessary to teach student nurses. It is not intended to replace graduate programs that focus on teaching registered nurses how to become effective clinical educators. Rather, the book's purpose is to simply serve as a complementary guide to providing effective clinical nursing instruction. This book is especially intended to assist those who have transitioned from the practice role to that of educator, offering them some advice and structure relating to the clinical instructor role.

Parts and Chapters

Part I includes Chapters 1, 2, and 3, and is an introduction to the clinical instructor's role. Chapter 1 presents the basic facts of clinical teaching and includes the expectations for many experienced and novice instructors. In this chapter, you are asked to assess your knowledge of this challenging role. Chapter 2 asks readers to assess their basic knowledge of standard rules and policies in nursing education. The chapter also shares information regarding the increased requirements dictated by hospitals prior to entry into the facility. There is an increased pace that all new instructors must keep up with. Advances in technology and informatics has led to nursing program websites that house course syllabi and nursing handbooks. Access to hospital documentation systems is dependent upon meeting various hospital requirements. Faculty are required to complete various online training for the schools and the various agencies. All of this training keeps clinical instructors very busy prior to the start of the clinical practicum! Chapter 3 titled "Your New World: Clinical Sites, Clinical Specialties, Clinical Students," differentiates the opportunities and challenges posed by various types of clinical sites and the variety of requirements dictated by the site and course specialty.

Part II focuses on the clinical teaching workload. Chapter 4 reviews the priority tasks for the clinical instructor as he or she works not only with students, but also with a variety of staff. This chapter highlights major responsibilities that will enhance the instructor's relationships with the staff and his or her students. The chapter also includes a survey of staff nurses, care technicians, and nurse managers regarding their expectations of clinical instructors. Chapter 5 highlights the orientation day and provides a sample template for that day. The orientation day is a key time for communication between the instructor and the students. Tips for fostering student independence and the utilization of a unit "scavenger hunt" are discussed. Chapter 6 addresses the challenges clinical faculty have in making sure students in the clinical setting fully understand the meaning of maintaining confidentiality of patient information and the many risk factors that can lead to potential violations.

Part III offers several strategies for maximizing the limited observation and supervision time inherent in the clinical rotation world. That is why many instructors attempt to "see it early." Chapters 7 and 8 review characteristics of "high fliers" and "not-so-high fliers." High fliers are students who will pass the course and possibly receive a higher-than-average grade. The "not-so-high fliers" are those who may receive lower grades than most or are at risk for course failure. Strategies to create collaboration between each type of student are delineated, as well as a depiction of the "student's own words."

Part IV presents the key aspects of clinical evaluation. This part includes the triad of the students' self-evaluation, the professor/instructor's evaluation, and the student's evaluation of the instructor. Chapter 9 discusses the importance of student self-evaluation. Students should realize that self-evaluation is a responsibility they will carry into their professional lives as registered nurses. To assist instructors in becoming more efficient in evaluating students, "anecdotal notes" are highlighted. Anecdotal notes are being required by many schools; they are seen as a supportive document in the evaluation phase. Chapter 10 provides evidence to support a mid-term and final evaluation even if the clinical rotation is as brief as 4 days. Chapter 11 contains a more elaborate discussion of warning signs for students who are in danger of failing. Unsatisfactory performance behavior is identified in this chapter. Chapter 12 presents the most common grading systems used in nursing programs: letter/number, pass/fail, or satisfactory/unsatisfactory grading systems. In addition, this chapter presents tips on seeking support when students challenge instructors' grades and how instructors can protect themselves from complications.

To have an organized and well-planned clinical day requires much planning and management work on the part of clinical instructors. Part V addresses how to manage the actual clinical day from preconferences, postconferences, and any unplanned events that may happen in between. Chapter 13 addresses preconference time where most clinical instructors are now incorporating teaching and prioritizing nursing goals. Chapter 14 shares new ideas on what can be done at postconference time. Chapter 15 shares helpful guidelines for instructors as they assign patients to students to complete the nursing process. There are also insights that will prepare the clinical instructor for certain unplanned events such as lateness in student arrival or changes invoked by the unit or floor environment. Chapter 16 highlights alternative assignments. This chapter describes assignment ideas in the event of a student absence. Chapter 17 provides several examples of unsafe practice events because the authors believe this is a continuous challenge for all instructors.

Part VI describes how to gain and maintain satisfaction in the role. Chapter 18 contains a survey taken from senior nursing students within 1 month of graduating from a baccalaureate nursing program. The survey asked such questions as "What are the most important things that a clinical nursing instructor can share with you and teach you?" Chapter 19 is new and is titled "Take Time for Self-Care." This chapter stresses the importance of self-care and the role it plays in modeling the same for your students. It presents simple practices that can be incorporated into the clinical day and taught to patients. Lastly, Part VII contains Chapters 20 and 21. Chapter 20 discusses the responsibility of clinical instructors regarding writing letters of reference and the growing amount of time expected to fulfill this component of the job. Chapter 21 updates the current thinking about the utilization of the simulation lab in nursing curricula. This chapter describes simulation experiences and highlights thoughts from certain students about the value and balance of simulation and real clinical experiences.

Each chapter includes "Essential Facts," a feature that highlights key elements of the chapter. Some chapters also provide questionnaires or exercises for instructors to complete. These are intended to assist in the understanding of the clinical nursing instructor role. Finally, the appendices include several key items that will help prepare instructors for the role. Among them is a new one, "Appendix D—The Student Report Sheet." Items in the appendices are supplemental material for the experienced instructor; however, some novice instructors may find them to be more valuable, especially if they have yet to embark on their first clinical instructor assignment.

DYNAMICS OF CLINICAL INSTRUCTION

As you read each chapter, you will realize the respect the authors have for clinical instruction and the academic goal of providing quality nursing education to future nurses. It is a challenging task to educate a student nurse. We have attempted, in our own way, to provide you—the clinical instructor—with some information about the basic dynamics of clinical instruction. As mentioned earlier, we have years of experience in the role because we truly enjoy it!

You should have fun and be open to humor in the role. If you are relaxed, this will be conveyed to your students and will enhance their performance. Moreover, you will quickly realize that there are many surprises in the role. Some students will forward you a "thank you" card at the end of the practicum. Also, do not be surprised if they seek you out at graduation. They may invite you to the final year student dinner or the pinning ceremony. Student nurses will become indebted to you and will want to visit you even after graduation from the program. It is a remarkable reward to have that kind of effect on your students.

You have taken a very important step in your professional nursing career. The fact that you are reading this book shows that you are truly interested in becoming an effective and successful teacher. You have made a commitment to become one of those clinical instructors whose name will be remembered by tomorrow's nurses.

Reference

Grant, R. (2016, February 3). The U.S. is running out of nurses. *The Atlantic.* Retrieved from https://www.theatlantic.com/health/archive/2016/02/nursing-shortage/459741

I

Appreciating Your New Identity: From Caregiver to Educator

1

Developing a New Identity as a Clinical Nursing Instructor

Both novice and experienced nursing teachers need to modify their mindsets on many occasions. They need to shift their actions from the delivery of quality care of patients to the delivery of quality education to students who will one day provide patient care. This chapter introduces the "top 11" facts essential for clinical nursing instruction.

This chapter presents a questionnaire for your completion. After answering the questions, you will find explanatory information designed to enhance the development and refinement of your identity as a clinical nursing instructor.

In this chapter, you will learn:

- How to begin the transition from staff nurse to clinical nursing instructor
- The basic facts of clinical teaching

You have just begun a journey from staff nurse to clinical nursing instructor. Or, perhaps, you have been a nursing instructor who always felt the need for more information, more guidance, and more specific examples and plans to successfully instruct your students. Throughout this book, you will learn concrete and useful information that you can use immediately—even on the same day that you read it.

To begin, you should ask yourself two questions:

1. What may be required for my transition from staff nurse to clinical nursing instructor?
2. Which of the following facts do I feel are important?

QUESTIONNAIRE

Place a T for true or an F for false next to the following facts. Then, review the answers that follow the questionnaire.

_____ 1. I will need to prove my clinical competency on a daily basis.
_____ 2. I will contribute to the nursing profession.
_____ 3. I must be friends with my students.
_____ 4. My students must always like me.
_____ 5. The unit's staff nurses and aides should be happy to take guidance from me.
_____ 6. I want to be familiar with the unit and the staff before I bring my students to the clinical setting.
_____ 7. I must know every detail about every patient that my students care for.
_____ 8. I must supervise every procedure and almost all interactions between my students and patients.
_____ 9. I will earn much more money in this position.
_____ 10. All of my students will be motivated to learn as much as possible.
_____ 11. I do not need to prepare for any simulation experiences with my students.

ANSWERS TO THE QUESTIONS: TRUE OR FALSE?

1. *I will need to prove my clinical competency on a daily basis.*
   False. Some of you are transitioning from practice as expert staff nurses. Others are tenured professors, academic experts who need additional guidance in supervising students and in grasping the many facets of clinical instruction. Whatever your background, the first item for a clinical instructor to remember is that you will have to supervise clinical experiences with student nurses. The students you will encounter, whether in 2- or 4-year programs, are novice learners. Learning to refrain from

performing any nursing skill or procedure for the student learner will be a major challenge. If the student is having a problem performing a basic clean dressing change on a wound, for example, you may be tempted to take over and complete the procedure. Resist taking over! Many seasoned clinical instructors will tell you, "Think more like a teacher and less like a nurse!" Your own professional goals of clinical competence should be tempered. Keep in mind that your role in the clinical setting is to enhance student learning by supervising (and not performing) skills. This involves using teaching and learning strategies to enable the student to perform the clinical skill with knowledge and eventual competence.

An effective clinical instructor uses these strategies, such as "questioning," "role-playing," and "interactive discussion," to improve students' thinking and problem-solving skills. This is not an easy task. Being a good teacher requires much practice and learning.

Essential Facts

With your students, think of yourself as a clinical teacher rather than a caregiver.

2. *I will contribute to the nursing profession.*

True. Many nurses become clinical instructors after realizing that they already have been contributing to advancing academic goals by assisting student nurses who have clinical rotations on their floor. Or some nurses may serve as "preceptors." Many schools have academic partnerships with hospitals, and the hospital nurses serve as preceptors who work side by side with student nurses. A student nurse may follow a preceptor's shift hours. This student–preceptor relationship is usually offered in independent course work, part of a scholars program, or embedded into a clinical practicum close to graduation. Many times, these preceptors offer to teach students because they themselves are taking graduate classes or hope to work in academia one day. Graduate education is the general preparation requirement for employment in most programs. However, state boards of nursing, school standards, and professional organizations can influence academic preparation requirements for employment (Penn, Dodge-Wilson, & Rosseter, 2008). Whether you are a part-time or full-time clinical instructor, you are contributing to a profession that is in great need of successful instructors who can teach students how to effectively care for their patients.

> **Essential Facts**
>
> The practice of clinical education is highly valued in this current environment of nursing shortages.

3. *I must be friends with my students.*

   False. If you go into clinical teaching thinking that you can be "friends" with your students, then your tenure in this role will be short. As a result of the combined objective and subjective nature of clinical instruction and evaluation, friendships with your students can lead to difficult situations, particularly during evaluation periods. Remember that each school's curriculum establishes many clinical objectives. If you share outside activities with students, you will expend energy that should be focused elsewhere—energy that should be used to enhance your students' clinical competence and help them meet clinical objectives. In the unfortunate event that you may have to discipline or correct a student under your tutelage, it will be more difficult if you have not maintained the "boundary of teacher : student." Keep personal information about yourself to a minimum.

> **Essential Facts**
>
> - Maintain the boundary of teacher : student.
> - Keep personal information out of the clinical setting.

4. *My students must always like me.*

   False. Face it, we all want to be liked as teachers. However, stay away from focusing on whether students "like" or "dislike" you. Clinical instructors may be so focused on this that they forget the main goals and objectives of the course they are teaching. You should focus primarily on the clinical objectives for your students and place less emphasis on whether students like, or even appreciate, your efforts. Don't get stuck on a student who dislikes you and is not as friendly or "warm" as your other students. This may be upsetting and cause emotional stress and worry that can affect your teaching and attitude toward your clinical group. Wouldn't you rather be the teacher who instills a memorable learning experience? Focus instead on the "aha" moments of your students—moments when your clinical thinking questions led to further student inquiry and successful application of concepts. Once you experience these moments, you will be hooked on teaching. Feelings of accomplishment is positive energy and much better for your emotional happiness then worrying about being "liked" or "disliked."

5. *The unit's staff nurses and aides should be happy to take guidance from me.*
   False. Staff personnel, nurses, and aides are familiar with required routines at their clinical agencies and are knowledgeable about their work. Although they are not happy about changes in policy or procedures, they will adapt in time. Thus, they will eventually accept you and your students and be willing to alter their routines a bit. However, they will not be receptive to verbal direction or recommendations from a clinical instructor. If you want to communicate with the staff, ask the nurse manager for the proper procedure.

   If, however, a staff member "corrects" you or a conflict develops, try to resolve the issue professionally. Although staff nurses also model professional behavior, you are the daily role model for your students. Remember this when you observe a procedure that is being done incorrectly and you want to provide input based on your practice experience. Recall that you are first a teacher and second a nurse. For those new to the clinical instructor role, this is one of the hardest lessons to learn.

   Your major goal as a clinical instructor is to teach your students. You are not there to teach the nurses or ancillary staff! If you do so, your energy is being misdirected. Instead, direct all your energy to your students. You need some degree of humility. Your goal is to facilitate communication among staff and students, so steer clear of any conflicts. Rather, focus on teaching and preparing your students for success in the practice arena.

> **Essential Facts**
>
> You are not there to teach the nurses or ancillary staff.

6. *I want to be familiar with the unit and the staff before I bring my students to the clinical setting.*

    True. It is often a prudent practice to go for a "trial run" before you drive to an unfamiliar spot. For example, many people drive to the location of a job interview a day or two in advance to make sure that they know of any detours or potential problems on the route. Similarly, it is vital for any instructor, whether new or familiar with the hospital unit, to visit the unit before the first clinical orientation day with the students. Call the nurse manager and arrange to visit for at least half a day. The nurse manager may meet with you for a brief period, during which you should be prepared to explain the clinical objectives of the course and provide the names of the students with the assigned clinical hours for the term or semester. Also be prepared to ask questions. It is his or her "turf!" You are a guest! Remember that!

    You may want to go through a "full shift" with a willing, veteran nurse, thereby becoming familiar with the "culture" and routines of the unit. The bonus is clear: You will have an experienced nurse ally waiting for you when you return with your students.

> **Essential Facts**
>
> Familiarity with the hospital unit and its staff is an essential element for student learning.

7. *I must know every detail about every patient that my students care for.*

    False. Remember that the staff nurse is ultimately responsible for the patients, not you! You need to know times of medications, safety information like "code status," NPO (nothing by mouth) status, necessary lab specimens, general diagnoses, and precautions, such as isolation standards. You cannot know all there is to know about the 10 or more patients being seen by the seven or eight students in your group.

Encourage your *students* to assume the responsibility for learning about their patients. It is the student who needs to feel the "pressure" of the obligation to thoroughly read the nursing documentation forms and to check with the primary nurse about the patient. Your job is to foster and encourage the student to gather the patient information and remember it throughout the clinical day.

Essential Facts

Encourage students to be responsible by having them thoroughly review each patient's chart, medication list, and care plan.

8. *I must supervise every procedure and almost all interactions between my students and patients.*

    False. You will be setting yourself up for failure and frustration very quickly if you try to practice this philosophy. Although you will need to supervise most medication administration, intravenous medication responsibilities, and new procedures (e.g., insertion of a urinary Foley catheter, insertion of a nasogastric tube, changing of a sterile dressing), you cannot be everywhere all of the time.

    In fact, depending on your schedule, you may sometimes allow the staff nurse to supervise your student in putting in a urinary Foley catheter or changing a sterile dressing. For example, you may be supervising one student's administration of intravenous medications when you are notified that another student needs to insert a urinary catheter immediately. If you have established a rapport with the primary nurse, whom you believe to be trustworthy and professional, and he or she offers to supervise your student, allow it to happen. You need to trust the staff nurses while broadening your students' experiences.

Essential Facts

Do not expect to see and supervise each student task.

9. I will earn much more money in this position.

   False. You may very likely earn less money initially than your graduating seniors do. This is not a lucrative field, except in the area of satisfaction. As we mentioned earlier, when one of your students has that "aha" moment, it will be worth the pay cut. Remember also that you will be working an academic year, with academic appointments for possibly 8 or 10 months. You will have opportunities to teach in the summer and develop new courses, which can boost your finances and your self-esteem. You may also be offered to teach in the classroom or help out in the lab. If you choose to seek a tenure-track full-time appointment, your salary will increase incrementally and possibly more quickly. If you work in an academic institution that has union representation for its professors, this is more likely to be true.

   Many opportunities exist to increase your income. You can publish, work as a staff nurse during periods off, consult, and work part time for one clinical rotation in a different nursing school. All of these expand your horizons. This is an important judgment call for you.

Essential Facts

Financial gain should not motivate you to become a clinical instructor. Rather, your motive should be to skillfully and effectively teach students to be successful nurses.

10. *All of my students will be motivated to learn as much as possible.*

    False. Sad to say, this is not always the case. Some students will have other life issues that interfere with their ability to devote the time and energy needed to a clinical nursing rotation. Others may not have realized what "nursing" really encompasses and may stay in the major just to graduate and get a job. These students, however, will be in the minority. You will receive satisfaction from the wonderful students who truly are motivated to learn and who will work extremely hard under your guidance. They are the future nurses of whom you will be proud and who will make teaching worthwhile for you. There is no greater satisfaction than to realize that your former students are surpassing you in knowledge—that they have become nurses whom you would want to care for you and for your family.

Essential Facts

You are helping to educate nurses whom you would want to care for you and your family.

11. *I do not need to prepare for any simulation experiences with my students.*
    False. The majority of nursing programs have simulation experiences integrated for all levels of the student learner. Associate and baccalaureate degree programs are using simulation in nursing schools to supplement clinical experiences and to apply didactic instruction just like the traditional clinical experiences. Simulation scenarios are being mapped to course, lab, and clinical objectives of most nursing programs. Clinical faculty will be exposed to this teaching strategy, and thus they will need to understand this very important instructional method. See Chapter 21 for further explanation of simulation experiences in clinical education.

Essential Facts

Be aware of the simulation experiences available for nursing students in various types of nursing programs.

This chapter begins to expose the nurse from the clinical practice setting to the many facets of being an educator in clinical education. The role of the practicing staff nurse is complex and full of daily challenges. The transition from practicing nurse to the academic world, supervising and teaching students, is equally challenging with dynamic issues that involve agencies, student policies, and patient care. These issues are tackled by having specific information that may be explicit and readily available to the teacher, but more often, information is lacking and gaps remain. Many seasoned educators (including the authors) continue to believe there are not enough resources and support for practicing nurses when they face this transition. Gaps with information still remain. This chapter and this book is a start toward bridging that gap, to serve as a resource in supporting nurses who have begun to embrace the clinical faculty role in academia.

Reference

Penn, B. K., Dodge-Wilson, L., & Rosseter, R. (2008). Transitioning from nursing practice to the teaching role. *The Online Journal of Issues in Nursing*, *13*(3), 1–14. doi:10.3912/OJIN.Vol13No03Man03

2

Understand the Rules: What Every Nursing Instructor Needs to Know About the Nursing Program's Policies

This chapter discusses the importance of the academic policies in the clinical setting and the specific information that will prove useful to the clinical instructor. The discussion emphasizes that the clinical instructor is responsible for enforcing these policies among his or her students. The chapter begins with a true/false exercise that will enable you to review your baseline knowledge about clinical instruction.

In this chapter, you will learn:

- Key tasks to be completed by the clinical instructor prior to starting the clinical practicum with students
- Information that is key to the success of the clinical instructor

KNOW YOUR BASELINE

Start by answering the true/false questions in Exhibit 2.1. Remember that all clinical instructors must complete a comprehensive examination of their school's nursing program before actually starting the clinical days with students. Thus, there is much preparation work for

Exhibit 2.1

True/False Exercise

For each statement, check either true or false.

True   False

_____ _____ 1. Clinical teaching involves no advance preparation.

_____ _____ 2. Familiarity with the nursing program is a priority before your first clinical day with students.

_____ _____ 3. The student handbook is one of the most important resources for all clinical instructors.

_____ _____ 4. Policies of academic work are not usually found in the student handbook.

_____ _____ 5. At the time of hire, you should expect to receive online and written materials about the nursing program.

Answers: 1. False; 2. True; 3. True; 4. False; 5. True

---

you as a clinical instructor before actually meeting your students! After signing your contract for employment, you will need to get access to campus e-mail and complete the training for your role. This training will be centered on informatics and technology. You will have to sign up for training to access the online learning management systems and learn to use the e-mail system that the school provides. Most schools frown on communicating with students using personal e-mail accounts. They have policies for e-mail accounts and will share these details with you.

EXPECTATIONS FOR NEW HIRES

According to Frances Amorin (personal communication, April 19, 2016), the Clinical Coordinator for clinical faculty at the College of Nursing, Villanova University, there are many items to collect from new hires. See the list she has compiled in Exhibit 2.2, her expectations for new clinical instructors.

Many of the items on this list are requirements of hospitals or clinical agencies. Part-time clinical faculty members have a certain number

Exhibit 2.2

Items to Collect From New Clinical Instructor Hires

- Online application and curriculum vitae
- Faculty information sheet
- Transcripts—undergraduate and graduate
- Form I-9—statement of immigration status; Form W-4
- Two letters of reference; current RN license
- Current cardiopulmonary resuscitation (CPR) card
- Current evidence of liability
- Evidence of medical insurance coverage
- State Board of Nursing form
- Child Abuse History clearance
- Criminal background check
- Fingerprints
- Current immunizations including measles, mumps, rubella, varicella, hepatitis B, Tdap, purified protein derivative (PPD) for tuberculosis, seasonal flu vaccine

Source: Courtesy of Frances Amorin.

---

of contracted days that they need to commit to as part of their agreement with the institution. Clinical instructors are expected to become somewhat familiar with the unit that they will be teaching before their first contact with their students. Required knowledge for clinical instructors includes, for example, the electronic medical record, the medication system, the type of patients, and the coordinating classroom content for the course that they will teach. Most schools provide faculty members with an online copy of the course syllabus. At times, a school will connect a new faculty member to another faculty member who is familiar with a certain clinical agency and who can acquaint the new instructor with important ground rules of that hospital or agency.

Also, early identification of any need for student remediation is paramount to enhance the opportunity for each student to be successful. In addition, "anecdotal notes" need to be completed by each instructor in order to complete the school's clinical evaluation and record any potential issues. See Chapter 10 for more guidelines on anecdotal notes.

In Exhibit 2.2, "current evidence of liability" is listed. This list is taken from a school in Pennsylvania. Please note that not all schools require this item or many of the items on this list. It is best for a clinical instructor to check with the appropriate state board of nursing to identify the specifics of liability when you are teaching. Not all state boards and nurse practice acts are consistent in their language regarding the true autonomy of the practicing student. Yes, your students do have liability insurance, but you too may be considered liable if the aforementioned standards are not in place when your student performs an unsafe act. As an instructor, it is prudent to carry liability insurance. Check with national nursing organizations, which can provide further information about liability insurance for educators. You can also check with the resource persons at your school program for this information.

At the time of hire, you will be given access to any training needed for success in the role. These are some of the materials you will receive or have access to:

- Requirements
  - Training for learning management system and school e-mail account access
  - Online requirements for entry into the agency (clinical practicum site)
- Essential clinical materials
  - Clinical course syllabus
  - Clinical practicum or academic calendar schedule
  - Clinical assignment sheet
  - Clinical evaluation tool (student and clinical faculty)
  - Diagnostic medication and calculation quiz (a sample copy)
- Faculty handbook/manual
  - Clinical job responsibilities
- Student handbook—clinical policies
  - Program goals
  - Dress code policy
  - Attendance policy
  - Safe/unsafe practice policy
  - Substance abuse or impaired student policy

By the time the instructor is hired, the nursing program chairperson or course coordinator (or designate) will probably have provided a clinical packet that contains essential materials, such as a course syllabus, faculty handbook, and student handbook. The instructor is expected to study these materials and return with any questions. Just as a hospital has ground rules and entry requirements that you need to understand, schools also have basic requirements. At this time, most nursing programs have these materials uploaded in their online (classroom) learning management systems (such as Blackboard, MyLearning, Moodle, and Canvas). You as an instructor will need to be familiar with these online systems because they contain much course detail and helpful resources. In some schools, clinical instructors can have access to theory and lab lesson plans.

HOSPITAL ENTRY REQUIREMENTS

Hospitals have become quite prescriptive with school and clinical faculty requirements. These are being predicated on the laws and rules set by accreditation agencies. Hospitals and most health care agencies alike will dictate that each clinical faculty entering their agency will either need to (a) complete a hospital-based orientation, (b) submit immunization and other health requirements, and/or (c) contact the nurse manager of that hospital unit to make arrangements for unit orientation. Several documents also need to be submitted to the hospital prior to your orientation day with the students. These required documents are similar to what students are expected to submit for entry into clinical practica: CPR verification, health requirements, and a background check. In some nursing programs, clinical faculty are expected to upload these health requirements using Complio, a cloud-based document management system. Complio can enable secure interface of documents between individuals and institutions.

CLINICAL PACKET OF ESSENTIAL MATERIALS

The clinical packet is usually a folder of sheets or forms that may include the current course syllabus; an academic calendar or a written outline that highlights the dates of the practicum; and, ideally, certain helpful forms, such as a blank clinical assignment sheet or a copy of a medication calculation quiz. This packet of information often contains the "clinical evaluation tool" that is the main instrument used to evaluate each student. This clinical evaluation form is generally filed in the student's folder at the conclusion of the practicum. Be sure you understand how to use it. Most programs link their tools to their mission and philosophy or a conceptual framework. To ensure reliability, a course coordinator or resource person will be sure to extensively assist you in navigating the use of this tool. There are extensive guidelines and a rubric that correspond to their grading and evaluation system. You can conduct an online search for these clinical forms as most programs now have them uploaded to their nursing websites, accessible to the world-wide community. It is current practice for most nursing programs to offer what is typically called an "adjunct faculty orientation" module. This module will highlight relevant information about the nursing program, faculty and student policies, and other helpful learning modules embedded in an online virtual learning environment. Most modules are currently being offered as part of an online computer program or a hybrid, a combination of face-to-face instruction and online instruction.

Clinical Syllabus and Calendar

In the clinical packet with essential materials, you will find the clinical syllabus with course and clinical objectives plus the calendar detailing the clinical practicum. Know these documents well. Curricular programs may be tweaked from year to year or semester to semester, and this will be reflected in the syllabus. You may be a seasoned clinical faculty at the school but will see a change that will first be found in the syllabus. There may be times someone will forget to tell you that the first 2 days of the practicum will involve off-campus training—possibly at the hospital computer lab or at the computer labs on campus. The syllabus is the important contract detailing expectations of the student for the course. Be very familiar with this and, if you have questions, seek a faculty member to interpret and answer your questions.

FACULTY HANDBOOK

The faculty handbook clearly outlines your role and associated expectations. In some programs, the information is relayed electronically through e-mail or clearly identified in a job description and in the orientation information that highlights the faculty role. It is the duty of the clinical instructor to keep himself or herself informed about the student functions of the nursing program. Specific responsibilities and duties are clearly identified in a job description. Be familiar with what the nursing program expects of you. For example, are you expected at the monthly faculty meetings? Do peers visit and evaluate you? If so, how often? What is your responsibility with final course grades? Your program dean or chairperson should refer you to someone who can assist you in obtaining necessary information. Most programs have a primary faculty resource for the instructor; they are called a "level" or "course" coordinator. For example, for a pediatrics course with a related practicum, the pediatrics course coordinator will be assigned to work closely with the clinical faculty regarding student assignments and course requirements. Other programs identify one faculty resource for several clinical practicum courses.

In addition, there is a new member of the clinical coordination team. Most nursing programs have now hired clinical coordinators to further enhance clinical practice coordination among all nursing course coordinators. This person is a full-time faculty member with relevant experience who may hold a graduate degree in nursing. The clinical coordinator will facilitate communication with the hospitals or health care agencies working with the nursing program. He or she will provide the clinical packet of information, can assist you in interpreting the clinical evaluation tool, and can inform you of any new program updates or changes.

STUDENT HANDBOOK

Of all the resources the clinical instructor receives, the student handbook is probably the most valuable and important. In most nursing programs, a student handbook is developed by the faculty in cooperation with students in that program. It is an outstanding resource for all clinical instructors, primarily because it spells out the policies and procedures relating to academic student work. In addition, the handbook contains information about the nursing program and curriculum. Thus, the student handbook has to provide specific details on both course and clinical requirements. It describes not only the program's policies, but also its mission, philosophy, and main goals, as required by accrediting bodies.

Program Goals

Clinical instructors are encouraged to understand the school's goals for its students. In a 4-year nursing program, for example, basic expectations for the second-year student will be different from those for the third-year or fourth-year student. In addition, each clinical site has setting-specific rules and policies; that is, the policies and procedures for a medical–surgical setting will be different from those in the community health clinical rotation. Students will usually receive this information from their clinical instructor at orientation or on their first day at the facility. There may be times when you are asked to share information about your school with others. For example, patients or hospital staff may be curious about the school's general program and policies. However, the most important reason to carefully examine the handbook is that it contains explicit instructions for the clinical aspects of the program.

Dress and Attendance Policies

Most health care agencies have policies on everything from dress codes to continuing attendance education. Familiarize yourself with the school's policies because you will be required to enforce them at the clinical site. One that you will need to enforce every day is the dress code! Students must adhere to this dress code, which is usually carefully monitored and evaluated. This code may specify attire, jewelry limitations, hair and nail length, facial piercing, hair color, and other aspects of one's appearance. Adherence to the dress code is identified in a student's clinical evaluation under objectives that specify "professional behavior."

The student handbook also identifies policies on absences, tardiness, and clinical practice expectations. There is usually a zero tolerance for absences or tardiness. Each and every clinical day is considered vital to the overall program. Lateness for the clinical day is always frowned upon. Tardiness and absences are further discussed in Chapter 15.

As mentioned earlier, health care agencies such as hospitals are starting to dictate requirements for clinical faculty that enter their facility. Please check with your hospital site about their specific dress code requirements for faculty. In general, most hospitals prefer clinical instructors to have white lab coats over business attire. For security purposes, they may also require the students and the faculty to wear a hospital-approved identification badge visibly when on their premises.

Safe/Unsafe Practice Policy

This policy usually involves only students majoring in nursing. Because of the nature of the nursing field, the practice setting can lead to an array of issues and potential unsafe incidents that may arise, especially with students who are novices to the various learning environments, multiple personnel, and changing patient conditions. This is an important policy that is usually addressed in detail by most schools. In some handbooks, "unsafe" practice may be defined as not being able to apply the nursing process. Patterns of unsafe practice are the most egregious because these may warrant dismissal from an academic program. "Anecdotal notes" as well as any meetings or conference time with the student must be clearly written with dates and times of incidents and action plans for students.

Substance Abuse or Impaired Student Policy

In most institutions, this policy is linked to the institutional handbook and policy on the use of drugs and alcohol in the clinical field. This policy is carefully reviewed with input from the lawyer affiliated with the main institution or college. The policy defines important concepts and clearly identifies what will happen to the student if a violation does occur. This is a clear and explicitly written policy is most schools.

In conclusion, not all of the policies encompassed by a nursing program have been identified here in this chapter. They are just too numerous to list. Many nursing programs now have their student nursing handbooks published and readily accessible on their websites. Take the time to look up some of these policies. Of course, some programs provide more and some provide less information in their student handbooks. Once you have done the necessary training and review of student handbooks, you will be ready to start focusing on preparing your students for the clinical practicum.

CLINICAL PRACTICUM

Exhibit 2.3 is an example of a checklist that will help guide you to what must be done before the *first day* of the clinical practicum. Chapter 3 provides an outline of the necessary and general information that must be shared with students on orientation day.

Yes, most clinical instructors agree that the student handbook is the first item to be reviewed, as it is usually considered the "bible." The novice instructor will probably focus initially on his or her job responsibilities, but the expert will quickly find and read the handbook. To begin the clinical rotation with students and to start planning

Exhibit 2.3

Instructor's Checklist

1. Understand job responsibilities
2. Familiarize yourself with the handbooks: student and faculty
   - Read the basic policies and procedures
3. Visit the agency
   - Meet with the nurse manager
   - Tour the unit
   - Meet with the staff personnel
4. Obtain access
   - Nursing program's online learning management system
   - Agency computers
   - Medication systems (Pyxis)
   - Electronic documentation systems

learning experiences and activities for them, the instructor needs a basic understanding of the school and its student policies. The student handbook is a solid starting place for that information.

Essential Facts

- Before the clinical practicum begins, make contact with your faculty resource.
- Understand the nursing program's goals and curriculum as highlighted in the student handbook.
- Before orientation day with students, have a clear understanding of the student policies applicable to your clinical course.

3

Your New World: Clinical Sites, Clinical Specialties, Clinical Students

In setting your personal goals as a clinical instructor, it is useful to develop your expectations with an understanding of the environment you will be working in. No two clinical experiences are completely alike. They will vary somewhat based on where they occur, the specialty they cover, and the composition of the student group assigned to that rotation.

In this chapter, you will learn:

- The differences in teaching clinical nursing students in pediatrics, maternity, medical–surgical, community health, and psychiatric–mental health as cited by practice experts
- The role of the clinical coordinator or course coordinator, who often is your first contact in a school of nursing
- The differences in teaching generic/traditional students (i.e., recent high school graduates) versus second-career students (i.e., older, work-experienced, pursuing second degrees)
- The differences in teaching today's generations in all programs
- The essential role of the group dynamics of your clinical group and how handling the dynamic can "make or break" a clinical experience

CLINICAL SITES AND SPECIALTIES

Many aspects of clinical teaching—and indeed any type of teaching—are universal. The teacher's expertise, appropriate preparation, an atmosphere conducive to motivated learning, clear communication between students and teachers, careful monitoring of student performance, and remediation as needed are all essential to a positive outcome. Clinical nursing instructors have an opportunity to build upon this time-tested template by placing these standard elements of teaching success within the context of the working environment. Specifically, giving some forethought to special considerations prompted by the location of the clinical site, the specialty being presented, and the readiness of the students to leverage their real-world exposure in acquiring actual nursing skills can move the needle from a good clinical experience to a great one. Following are the insights of seasoned clinical nursing instructors as they share their own thoughts regarding both the fundamentals of clinical teaching as well as personal insights concerning their own particular specialties.

Pediatrics
Michelle M. Kelly, PhD, CRNP

In pediatrics, as in other specialties, the instructor is responsible for the student and the patient. Unlike adult specialties, however, the family plays a much larger role in the equation. Parents, when present, are the voice of the patient and a critical part of the care team. When students enter the room for the first time, they are focused on the child, focused on the task at hand. Instructors often find themselves speaking with the parents while simultaneously watching the skills or assessment being performed. As pediatric nurses we do this together—talk to the child and the parent(s), and accomplish the task at hand. Students need time to develop that ability, and instructors may model that behavior for the student.

The other large component of pediatrics is an appreciation and understanding of the developmental stage of the patient being cared for by the student. Adults are adults, and children may be infants, toddlers, preschool age, school age, or adolescents. The children may be all on the same unit at the same time. The days of cohorting children by age are gone in most facilities. Instead, we cohort by medical condition, specialty, or acuity. This means that the instructor must have a strong background in normal developmental and behavioral stages in order to share this with students. And then we must face the variations in developmental stages due to developmental delay, as well as the transient alterations due to illness or injury. These challenges, which may have arisen from altered expectations of developmental abilities, may lead to robust postconference discussions.

A pediatric instructor must be someone with a strong background in pediatrics and a compassion for students. Flexibility and a strong pediatric skill set are also very important. Students look to undergraduate instructors as leaders and mentors, so instructors should be active in their profession, maintain a current evidence-based practice skill set, and be seen as clinical experts. Actively practicing instructors are the ideal, but full-time faculty may have difficulty maintaining an active clinical practice as well as a full teaching load.

The best part of being a clinical instructor is watching a student evolve from frightened student to competent novice. You need to teach students to believe in themselves, to ask questions in a safe environment, and to advocate for their patients. Another joy is knowing that you modeled positive interactions between yourself and students, watching tradition passed on to the next generation of students. Perhaps the best way to see this is when you return to a nursing unit to find a former student precepting a current student, or when a former student joins your teaching group as a clinical instructor.

Challenging students, either those who display repeated subpar skill mastery or those whose demeanor precludes their successful transition to a novice nurse, are the bane of all nursing instructors. I recall a student who displayed true arrogance, with disregard for both procedures and the role of a student. The student was providing suboptimal care—not truly dangerous, but far below the standards set by the university. When addressed, the student was flippant and disruptive during postconferences. To compound the issue, previous instructors had a dissimilar experience with the student, who earned good grades and high marks in clinical work. As an adjunct clinical faculty, I felt somewhat adrift and not sure how to handle the student or her looming failure in the course. I reached out to the course leader, who met with the student and myself to discuss her performance on campus away from the clinical setting. We were able to have the student spend two clinical days with a different instructor who had a clinical group at the same hospital, just on a different unit. The second faculty member confirmed my assessment of the student and supported the failing clinical grade. If I had not reached out to the course leader, the opportunity to discuss and validate my assessment would have been lost. Instructors, many of whom are adjunct faculty, need to feel supported by the course leaders, clinical coordinators, and other university faculty.

Be an advocate for your students. Help them have experiences that will show them the joys, challenges, and wonders of being a nurse. Regulations and hospital restrictions preclude them from doing much of the care they will be expected to do as a nurse. Step in, offer to do the procedure or dressing change for the nurse so that your students can have a more detailed experience—even if they do not get to do it themselves. Advocate for the observational experience that puts students in the path of success and greatness, and that teaches them what the possibilities are.

Instill your passion for nursing in your students. Show them why you love doing what you do. Point out the bad examples, but do it in a way that says, as a nurse you can change this culture, you can improve outcomes, you can be an advocate for your patients. Be a role model. They are watching you. Do not check your phone every 5 minutes, do not answer emails while on the unit, do not take part in disparaging of coworkers or others. But show them you are human as well. Cry when a patient dies. Talk about it in postconference. Teach them that processing sadness is part of what we do and is just as important as sharing the joys.

Maternity
Katherine A. Conroy, MS, RN

In maternity, the student may be asked to deal with two distinct patients. The woman in labor is experiencing a normal development crisis of giving birth. She is a well woman. The role of the nurse is to closely monitor the woman and validate that she is physiologically within the norms of a healthy, normal labor. In addition, the nurse/student nurse:

- Assesses the psychological well being of the woman.
- Supports the woman as she copes with the changes that come with the stages of labor.
- Educates the woman about the labor process and reassure her about the normalcy of her labor.
- Supports the woman's choice of coping skills, offering other choices when her coping seems to be inadequate.

The education and the support skills offered by the nurse/student nurse include any person or persons designated by the woman as her support. In labor, there is always the possibility that the woman can deviate from the normal and quickly be in a physiological crisis. This nursing environment asks the nurse/student nurse to be alert to any deviation and to possess the skills needed when a crisis arises. Of course, always realize that there are two people she is caring for, woman and child in the womb.

The neonate is the second patient. At time of birth, the neonate must quickly adapt to extrauterine life. The nurse/student nurse assesses the signs of adaptation and supports the process as needed. Until recently, the focus was limited to the physiological adaptation. We, as health care providers, now recognize that keeping the infant with the mother (skin to skin on mother's chest for the first hour of life) addresses the psychological well-being of the mother and the infant. Since instituting the skin-to-skin practice, the majority of infants maintain their body temperature, blood sugar level, and have successful first breastfeedings. The nurse can do all needed assessments of the neonate while the neonate is on the mother's chest. Weights and measurements are deferred until later. The nurse/student nurse must know the norms for a neonate, which are very different from those for an adult. The neonate size leaves little margin for error when there is a deviation from the norm. For example, an infant who becomes hypothermic runs the risk of opening the newly closed foramen ovale, leading to metabolic acidosis. The neonate cannot communicate "not feeling well," and he or she is dependent on the caregiver to be observant and consistently mindful of safety issues at this age.

The postpartum woman is in need of physiological and psychological assessment as she begins to recover from birth. The nurse/student nurse assessments validate the normal processes of returning to the prepregnant state, especially relating to the uterus. It is necessary to provide education about what is normal during the 6 weeks of postpartum recovery. The nurse/student nurse helps support the woman as she assumes the role of mother and demonstrates and reinforces safe infant care.

Upon further reflection, I would contend that a third patient exists for the nurse/student nurse in maternity; that is the family, which is defined in a broad sense. The nurse/student nurse supports the family as a unit, reinforcing mothers, fathers, siblings, grandparents, and others (identified as family by the primary unit) as they adjust and expand in their role required by the addition of the neonate. Anticipatory guidance about such things as homecoming day can help with this adjustment.

The maternity clinical instructor must be knowledgeable in this area of practice and be enthusiastic about nursing. The instructor must be a clear communicator and be able to adjust the teaching to meet the level of students. The teacher needs to be respectful of students and clear about the expectations for student. The teacher must hold students accountable for their practice. The instructor must be approachable and open to questions, especially when supervising in the clinical area. The person should enjoy teaching. The patient's safety is first priority.

Maternity is usually a happy area but also a pivotal time in a woman's life. It offers an opportunity to support a woman both physically and mentally but also to empower her. When teaching students about maternity, you have the opportunity to discuss in postseminar a life experience their mothers had and perhaps a student has had or could have in the future. I think it can be a personal growth opportunity as a person observes and then reflects on childbirth without it being his or her personal experience.

As in other clinical areas, maternity is not without its challenges as the following account will illustrate. The policy at one particular hospital was "no nail polish or artificial nails." Students were told this in an on-campus orientation meeting. During the observational orientation day (no patient care by the students), I noticed a student had long nails with nail polish. I told the student she had to remove the nail polish and trim her nails and explained that the nails represented a risk for the neonate. The following week, the student arrived in the hospital with long, polished nails. I sent her home and she had a clinical absence. Nurses must be committed to patient safety.

Be aware of your own limitations as a clinical instructor. Only take clinical assignments for your students that you can safely supervise. Unless a formal arrangement is made with the nursing staff, the staff nurse a student reports to is not obliged to observe or validate the condition of the patient. The instructor is responsible to have received all the assessments from the students and direct their follow-up as needed. Ask for help from staff you have identified as being positive—both positive as nurses and toward students. Patient safety is foremost. Do not be afraid to ask questions about the nonformalized workings of the unit. You need to know the policies and procedures, but there are also less formal ways of doing things you need to know to ensure smooth working relationships among teachers, students, and staff. Be pleasant. Show interest in the staff as individuals but avoid unit politics. Construct any written assignment for the clinical course that will demonstrate an expected student outcome. Keep a clinical journal. Students, patients assigned, and outcomes for that day should be recorded before you leave the clinical site.

Medical–Surgical
Susan Stabler-Haas, PMHCNS-BC, RN

In teaching medical–surgical, or med-surg, nursing, much depends on the level of the student for whom you are responsible before creating your level of expectations. For example, if students are in their first clinical situation in med–surg, you must start out with teaching very basic patient care—as basic as how to introduce yourself to the patient and family, how to speak and get report, what to report to the primary nurse, and how to procure vital signs. Most students have had simulation lab experiences where they practice and learn these basic skills. This is helpful, but as the clinical instructor you still need to intensely observe your students while they operate in the real world of patient care.

Be sure to check the accuracy of your students' vital sign readings by taking a patient blood pressure immediately after they do, or simultaneously when a double stethoscope is available. Do not allow them to rely solely on electronic blood pressure measurements, because it is essential for them to develop the skill of taking blood pressure manually. There can be quite a difference in taking a blood pressure on an elderly 90-pound patient versus that of a manikin in the simulation lab. Given the varied patients, varied diagnoses, and varied intensity of illness each med–surg experience brings, the med–surg clinical instructor must be very flexible in calmly balancing multiple needs at one time.

The successful instructor will also communicate well with staff and students alike. Diane Ellis (MSN, RN, CCRN) is a university med-surg program coordinator who stresses the importance of instructor-student communication at the med–surg clinical site in this way: "Give feedback often and a give a lot of it. Provide written expectations at midterm to student. Explain clearly what they need to do to get an 'A.' Tell them to come to you and share thoughts and ideas. If they share their thinking then you know they are connecting the dots" (personal communication, November 18, 2016).

Be pleasant and cordial with your med–surg students but remember that your relationship with them is that of a teacher and mentor, not a friend. Above all, be fair in your dealings with them. Some useful "rules of the road" are succinctly captured in an intriguing webinar presentation called "Creating a Fair and Just Culture Within Schools of Nursing" by Barnsteiner and Disch (2016). Here are these rules:

- Students need to feel as accountable for, and prepared to, contribute to a safe environment as for delivering quality nursing care.
- Mistakes are part of learning and professional practice.

- Students should be held accountable for their actions, but not blamed for system faults beyond their control.
- Students who act recklessly may need to fail the course or be dismissed from the program.

The importance of holding students accountable cannot be overemphasized. One illustration of this vital aspect of the instructor role need revolves around medication administration. There are many clinical areas now in which students are not permitted to administer medications. When this valuable learning opportunity is permitted, it often falls to the med–surg instructor to supervise the student medication administration experience. This is quite a challenging role. Once I had a student who was assigned to give medications and thus was required to have knowledge about the assigned drugs that would be given that day. Unfortunately, soon after the student announced that she was ready to give medications, it became apparent that she did not know anything about them even though she had access to the hospital's easy-to-use online medication reference system. The administration of medications took an inordinately long time and a patient needed to leave the unit before all of the medications were given. I told the student to summon me when the patient returned to the floor so the medication administration process could continue. Later that morning when I saw the student, I learned that she had just given the remaining medications on her own. There was no remorse or anxiety expressed by the student, who merely said, "I thought it would be okay." In this incident, I was supported by the course coordinator to document the incident and document how she could successfully meet the objectives of the course during her next opportunity to administer medications. The student was further informed that she was in jeopardy of failing the course if the behavior was repeated. Most hospitals and nursing facilities now have it documented in their clinical faculty expectations that nursing instructors must supervise all medication administration to their patients.

Despite your strong background in med–surg and possibly critical care, you as the instructor will not always know all of the answers to the questions suddenly posed by students. As such, you must be willing to ask questions and also research medications on the unit as needed. Determine which nurse on the unit is a safe and skilled practitioner and use that person as a resource for your questions. Rather than feeling embarrassed by a knowledge gap of your own, seize upon it as a chance to role-model what a nurse should do when this inevitable situation presents itself. When you do not know something about a particular diagnosis, medication, or procedure, be truthful. In doing so you will show yourself as being authentic, and your students will appreciate you for it. In that same role-modeling vein, it is helpful for your students to see you enjoying your own role as a nurse. Try to find time to converse with a patient, perform assessment skills, assist with bathing, or give a back rub.

By the end of the rotation, you should have a sense of accomplishment in that you were able to acquaint your nursing novices with the risks and rewards of their chosen profession. Remembering that first clinical day when the students were afraid to touch a patient and watching them on the last day as they manage two or three at a time may bring a smile. It will also be gratifying to listen in postconferences as the students begin to assimilate classroom and clinical knowledge—realizing that they actually do know something about being a nurse. You will have that same sense of pride when the patient your student has just cared for compliments him or her and requests to have that same student the next clinical day. Even after the clinical rotation has ended, getting e-mails and notes from graduates that you have taught can be meaningful. A simple note from them informing you that they are in a new registered nursing position and how grateful they are to you in helping them get there will remind you why you decided to teach nursing.

Community Health
Kathleen Williams Yates, MSN, RN

In the community health setting, the role of the instructor extends from supervising to advising. When the students are going out into the community on home health visits, the instructor cannot be with all of the students at various homes at the same time. The students visit together in pairs at patients' homes. The instructor usually goes with one of these groups for evaluation purposes. The instructor also hosts preconferences and postconferences with the students at the home health agency. A preconference consists of gathering patient information and developing a plan together that the students will then implement. A postconference after the completed student visit consists of an evaluation of how the visit went, the plan for the next visit, documentation of visit outcomes, reporting to the primary nurse, and any questions or concerns. Because the instructor is not with the students personally for the majority of their home health visits, the instructor advises and collaborates with the students regarding patient care, assessments, implementation, and evaluation. Although the students perform their patient visits independently, they should always have access to immediate communication with the instructor, primary nurse, and home health agency.

In a community instructor, I look for an individual who is encouraging and able to instill a sense of confidence in his or her students. In the beginning of the rotation, the students usually need extra reassurance that they are capable and fully prepared to perform these visits in the home without being directly supervised.

I find teaching community nursing to be the most rewarding of all the nursing courses to instruct. It is the last course that the students take before they graduate, take NCLEX, and hopefully join the nursing profession. They come to this course with tremendous knowledge and excitement. In my opinion, to have the opportunity to collaborate with the students is the most satisfying aspect in teaching this course.

Of course, problems can occur. Once there was an incident with a group of students that made a visit to a patient who had an extremely high blood pressure. The students did not notify the instructor, nurse, doctor, or agency. They left the patient's home without a plan or intervention that needed to be implemented. When the students returned to the agency and reported the patient's status, I immediately went with them back to the home to reassess the patient. The patient did have a high blood pressure, and a 911 call was necessary. This was a learning experience for the students: Never leave an unstable patient. I now use this as a real-life example for all of my future clinical groups.

Instructing in the community health setting is quite different than in a hospital setting where you are able to directly oversee the students. It is difficult for a new community health instructor to "let go" and give the students autonomy. As educators, we need to be confident that they have been properly prepared and are capable of performing thorough and accurate nursing assessments and interventions without our supervision.

Psychiatric–Mental Health
Jessica Vann, MS, APRN, NP-C

In psychiatric/mental health nursing, the instructor is trying to get the students to be less task oriented and to focus on the patient as a whole. Previously, their focus was on caring for the patient's physical needs and although they might have been aware of an emotional need, they may have glossed over it. Now, we are asking them to address the patient's emotions directly and explore his or her feelings more deeply.

The successful instructor is someone who is patient and sensitive to the students' needs. Many students come to the psychiatric–mental health clinical rotation with apprehension and fear. The instructor needs to have the ability to allay those fears while managing his or her expectations. Calmly setting the stage for your students may even redirect the career interest of some to a field within nursing that they would otherwise never have considered. It is personally fulfilling when your students at least walk away from the experience with a newfound respect for this particular patient population and those that serve it.

Be cognizant of the potential for the psychiatric–mental health nursing clinical rotation to bring a student's own personal or family struggles to the surface. One student in particular acknowledged some psychiatric issues of her own and felt she had nothing to give to this population. It took a lot of coaching, counseling, and redirection but once the student realized what she had to offer, she excelled in the clinical setting and became one of my best students.

Use creative and innovative ways to get the students interested in psychiatric–mental health nursing. Also, realize that this role will often include being emotionally present for the students and the issues they are experiencing. Remember, it is okay to take a step back and collect yourself before dealing with student issues.

CLINICAL STUDENTS

Following are general characterizations, but the contrast is interesting to note nonetheless. It is beneficial for the clinical professor to be cognizant of the type of student to be taught—generic/traditional versus second career—to set the stage for successful interaction over the course of the rotation. This is true regardless of the type of nursing programs (i.e., diploma, 2-year associate degree, or 4-year baccalaureate).

Generic Nursing Students

The generic student is usually fresh out of high school, and nursing school is the first post–high school experience in his or her career pursuit. Generic students may require more detailed instructions than the second-career student described next. They may need you to explain in some detail what it means to do a self-evaluation (for a clinical rotation), because they have never had to do one for a job. Examples from previous students can help them understand what you want. You also may need to really emphasize if you want anything in a paper copy because their membership in the "digital native" generation commonly eschews the use of paper as a means of communication.

Generic students crave feedback. They have grown up in an era of remarkable connectedness. They are accustomed to receiving instantaneous reaction from parents, teachers, and coaches. They have grown accustomed to getting immediate response to questions and see no impediment to sharing their unsolicited opinions and commentary.

Second-Career (Second-Degree) Nursing Students

As the term implies, these students may have already received a college degree in another area of study or had a career in another field and now desire a nursing career. Not surprisingly, second-career/second-degree students tend to be older, already working in some capacity other than nursing, and more often than not paying for the education themselves. These students want notice of all assignments and requirements yesterday! They often have spouses and children, older parents requiring their attention, job demands, and a host of other personal obligations that must be balanced in order to accomplish the new goal of becoming a nurse. Although these factors can produce very motivated students who are a delight to teach, it can also yield dispirited and depleted candidates for nursing degrees. Managing the stress of this group can be one of the most difficult jobs in nursing. They may feel that any course grade below an "A" is a failure. Maybe the stakes are higher for the second-degree student. Maybe they feel that the decision to terminate their initial career choice now means that the decision to enter the nursing field must work out at all costs. Whatever the case, expect these older second-degree students to be somewhat intense.

As a clinical instructor teaching either the generic or second-degree students, you must have a firm sense of yourself. You must be comfortable saying to them, "I do not know, so would you please look it up" (or you, the instructor, looks it up). You are a role model who is teaching them that safe care does not mean you know all of the answers. Try not to take it personally if your expertise is challenged. Believe it or not, many of today's students will question your direction even if you have been in your field of expertise for many years. You may hear statements from them like, "I thought (or I read) that is not true." Take a deep breath and then ask them to provide the documentation to support their argument. In the unlikely event that this documentation shows them to be correct, acknowledge that fact. Clinical faculty and students have a common goal of safe patient care, and that requires humility and accepting that no one knows it all.

Clinical Group Dynamics

Ignore clinical group dynamics at your own peril! Surprisingly, little is written about this essential part of being a clinical instructor. Most clinical nursing groups consist of at least six to 10 students. Like the patient population that they will soon care for, the composition of the clinical group may represent an ever-changing blend of culture, gender, and ethnicity. All of these factors contribute to how your group will work together and function and learn. The degree of cohesiveness established within the clinical group will all affect your daily life.

Establishing rapport between yourself and the clinical group and among the members of the clinical group itself is a process that can be marked by the four distinct stages: pregroup, transition, working, and final (Corey, Corey, & Corey, 2010). Following are some considerations for your clinical group offered within the context of these four stages.

Pregroup Stage

Careful thought and attention must be given to your orientation day. Your students all have their own anxieties and concerns. Create an atmosphere where they feel safe to express them. For example, one student's father recently died from alcoholic cirrhosis and now will be with you in the clinical psychiatric–mental health rotation, where addiction issues are rampant. The way that you handle each student's question and issues will determine if the clinical group is a safe place to share concerns and to learn.

Transition Stage

This is the stage where students decide what they need help with regarding objectives, accept responsibility for their learning, and how they can assist each other.

Working Stage

This is the productive stage where students are administering medications and reviewing the problems they had with the clinical group. They are speaking about the difficulties they may have had with their primary nurse and the group can figure out how to handle the situation the next time. Sometimes, conflicts develop between you and one or more students or among the students. Students may say that you are not available when they need you, or that they cannot find you on the unit, and so on. Keep calm and do not become defensive. Help the students solve problems, entertain their suggestions, and also do not hesitate to inform them about the realities of your role and your time limitations with six to 10 or more students or with monitoring students on different units. Occasionally, students may harass or talk about a peer in conferences or "behind their backs." Address that immediately with each student, stating that incivility will not be tolerated. Remind them that the world of nursing consists of a myriad of personalities, and one of the essential attributes of a nurse is the ability to work alongside many different types of people.

At the same time, pay attention to any student who can "sabotage" your clinical group directly or indirectly. One member of a given clinical group may have a conflictual relationship with another member, and their animosity toward each other can easily precipitate a similar divide among the remaining students. Still others may have personality disorders or more latent issues that will be triggered by your authority as an instructor. Perhaps you remind them of a parent with whom they have a conflictual relationship. It is not uncommon for such students to unconsciously view you as a parental surrogate, causing them to redirect their anger toward you at the slightest provocation. When you observe a particular student whose demeanor poses a threat to clinical group harmony, seek support from your clinical coordinator early on. A private chat with the offending student may be sufficient to get things back on the proper track.

If the counseling session does not have the desired effect, document all pertinent facts to create an electronic trail. Unless school policy dictates otherwise, consider sharing the document with the recalcitrant student as a formal corrective action. More often than not, taking this step will lead to a chilling effect on the troubling behavior, while reinforcing your commitment to provide an atmosphere that is conducive to learning for all of your students. When all else fails, a meeting involving you, the student, the clinical coordinator, and any other appropriate representative of administration may be warranted to resolve the problem.

Final Stage

Identify what was learned and how this learning will continue to be retained as you progress in each nursing course. Identify as a group areas that they may need to review on their time. For example, if your students gave medications and had very little opportunity to give parenteral medications, have them go back to the lab or encourage them to identify this need at the beginning of their next rotation.

Most clinical groups are delightful, and you will enjoy much personal satisfaction in watching their development.

Essential Facts

- Although many aspects of clinical teaching are universal, differences in teaching clinical nursing students according to specialty do exist.
- The clinical coordinator is normally your first contact in a school of nursing.
- Generally speaking, there are differences in generic students (younger, recent high school graduates) and second-career students (older, working students, perhaps with a prior degree).
- Properly handling group dynamics can "make or break" a clinical experience.

References

Barnsteiner, J., & Disch, J. (2016). QSEN update: Creating a just culture within schools of nursing [webinar]. Retrieved from http://www.aacnnursing.org/Professional-Development/Webinar-Info/sessionaltcd/WFR16_03_31

Corey, M., Corey, G., & Corey, C. (2010). *Groups: Process and practice* (8th ed.). Belmont, CA: Brooks/Cole.

II

Your Success Depends on You: Preparing for Your Clinical Teaching Assignment

4

You Are a Guest, So Act Like One

Your success depends on you! This is the first chapter to discuss the essential and "lifesaving" relationship between the clinical instructor and the clinical unit staff. The unit to which you are assigned is *not* a classroom. It is the nursing staff's turf. You are a guest. This chapter provides two examples of novice instructors with different techniques in the clinical setting. You decide whose approach is the more effective and, therefore, the one you should adopt.

In this chapter, you will learn:

- The art of recognizing the expertise of each nurse and patient care technician (PCT) and how each one is an expert in his or her domain (even if you disagree with his or her actions)
- Information and using "EQ" (emotional intelligence quotient) can "make or break" a clinical instructor
- How to effectively interact with the nursing staff

The clinical site is not an alternative classroom, and it should not be considered the teacher's turf. The clinical site is a nursing unit and therefore the domain of the nurses who staff it. Your role as clinical instructor does not alter the fact that you are ultimately a guest on their floor or unit. Your goal is to establish the essential and professional "lifesaving" relationship between you and the unit's nursing staff.

The patients for whom the students will care are the responsibility of the unit's staff nurses and technicians. Accede to their sovereignty over patient care. Although rarely discussed in graduate school, this largely unspoken rule is integral to the success of the clinical nursing instructor. Always acknowledge the staff nurses as the experts in rendering care to their patients, even if circumstances may occasionally cause you to question that expertise. There are avenues you can follow if you feel it important to your students' or the patients' welfare to mention a unit nurse's behavior. First, discuss your concerns with the school's coordinator for the course. He or she may have had similar issues in a previous rotation and can give you the benefit of his or her prior experiences. Next, you may need to discuss your concerns with the nursing manager. A word of caution must be given here: Unless a patient's safety is threatened, as a new nursing instructor it is best to pause and seek guidance from either a more seasoned instructor or the school's coordinator before involving the unit's manager with a specific staff complaint. The importance of adopting the proper approach in relation to the nursing staff is illustrated in Exhibits 4.1 and 4.2, which offer two examples of nursing instructors who are about to bring their students into a new unit. You decide which instructor's approach is the more effective.

CASE STUDIES: INTRODUCING STUDENTS TO THE CLINICAL SETTING AND STAFF

Lessons Learned From the Case Studies

Based on these case studies, answer the following questions:

- Which nursing instructor will be successful?
- Which technique received the most positive reaction and feedback?
- Which students will have the best learning experience?
- Which instructor utilized "EQ?"

Unlike Bob, Mary clearly understood that she was a "guest" at the clinical site. She inquired about the agency and apprised the manager about the students' abilities. She asked the manager to assign nurses who really wanted to work with students, thus allowing the staff nurses to have input into the mentoring process. If the members of the nursing staff are given a choice and a voice in teaching (or not teaching) students, it will result in a better experience for the students—and the instructor.

Exhibit 4.1

Bob's Approach

Bob is a new hire, eager to begin his first position as a clinical nursing instructor. He has been a critical care nurse for the past 2 years and recently completed his master's degree. He is also new to the facility to which he will bring his first group of students and has called the nurse manager to arrange a meeting with her. He tells the manager that the students will take only patients who are oriented to person, place, and time, and who are able to communicate clearly. He also informs the manager that the students will *not* be helping the patients with their morning care or with any hygiene needs. Bob states, "The students are here to learn their future professional role and that does not include bed making and baths." The manager terminates the meeting abruptly and tells Bob that she thinks there may be a conflict with accommodating his students because a different school of nursing may also be scheduled for the same days. Bob is almost apoplectic, stammering that his students should have priority. The meeting ends badly.

Exhibit 4.2

Mary's Approach

Mary, who has two more courses to complete for her master's degree, has 5 years of experience as a home health nurse. She has taught clinical students before. Mary has gathered information about the home health agency to which she will soon be bringing her students and has arranged to meet with the nurse manager. Her students will be working with the agency's nurses and going on home visits with them. Mary explains the objectives of the nursing course to the nurse manager. She details her own experience and acquaints him with the level of expertise of her new students. She requests that the manager tell her which nurses would be most appropriate for the students to accompany on their home care visits. She stresses that the students are prepared to perform many functions under the direct supervision of the professional nurses with whom they are paired. Mary uses the meeting as an opportunity to compliment the nurse manager for allowing students to have this learning experience. Finally, Mary offers to join a nurse herself for one or two visits before the students begin their rotation, so that mutual expectations might be realistically set. The manager arranges for Mary to spend a half-day with one of her more experienced nurses and also states that he will discuss the students' impending arrival at the next agency staff meeting. When he meets with his staff, he intends to highlight the mutual benefits of this professional–student interaction and promises to call back with the names of the nurses who will mentor these students.

Mary also demonstrated her ability to utilize her EQ. EQ describes an ability or capacity to perceive, assess, and manage the emotions of oneself and of others (Goleman, 1995). She did independent research about the agency, discussed her own expertise and experience, sought the input of the manager, expressed her students' willingness to help the staff, complimented the unit's staff, and extended herself to work with the nurses, seeking their input. As you see in Exhibit 4.2, Mary included many of the provisions that the nursing staff stated were crucial for nursing instructors to be successful when surveyed.

In conclusion, the rewards from spending at least 1 day (often on your own time) in the new unit where you will be teaching student nurses far outweigh your time investment.

EFFECTIVE INTERACTION WITH THE NURSING STAFF

As is true in any human interaction, understanding the other person's perspective will enhance the chances of a successful outcome. Your hosts in the unit have their own perspectives in terms of their expectations of the clinical instructor and the nursing students. Failure to understand these expectations can lead the unit staff to conclude that you are not fulfilling your responsibility as a guest, even if the omission is quite innocent on your part. The key here is to communicate with the unit staff. So ask: What do they expect from you and the students? Honor their requests when reasonable, and explain the constraints when you and your charges cannot comply. Exhibit 4.3 provides input from two different nursing staffs regarding key questions.

Exhibit 4.3

Informal Survey of Nurses, Patient Care Technicians, and Nurse Managers

1. What are the most helpful things a clinical instructor can do?
   - Make a list of the students and the patients they are assigned to, and whether they are giving medications that day.
   - Advise the nurse of any issue or change in patient status.
   - Let nurses know what they can help students do.
   - Assign patients to students prior to the staff taking report.
   - Closely monitor the students to ensure that they are not just sitting around.

- Be present to answer student questions.
- Help students with medication passes.
- Be clear about what students are able to do, such as give medications, chart, and so on.
- Inform staff about the type of patients the clinical instructor is looking for.
- Closely monitor patients that the students are assigned to.
- Ask the patient care technician about the unit's morning care routine to avoid confusion.
- Do not allow students to sit in the conference room for most of the shift.

2. Upon arrival each day, what interaction of students with staff is appropriate?
   - Introduce themselves to the nurse and patient care technician with whom they will be working, and indicate what they plan to do (e.g., bath, medications, vital signs).
   - Give the nurses time to get report from the prior shift before posing questions.
   - Accompany the nurse on walking rounds if possible.
   - Review available information on the patient's prior night and goals for the day.
   - Introduce themselves to each new patient to whom they are assigned.
   - Determine whether patients need help eating and whether they are scheduled for tests that day.
   - Check the computer for orders.
   - Take the patient's vital signs in the first interaction.
   - As the day progresses, keep the nurse informed as to what they have done.

3. Upon leaving each day, what interaction of students with staff is appropriate? What should the students' final activities be?
   - Let the staff know when they are done for the day.
   - Do a final set of vital signs before leaving.
   - Give a report of pertinent information, including significant findings and concerns.
   - Document intakes and outputs.
   - Let the nurses and patient care technicians know what was and was not done.
   - Do not forget to say good-bye to the patients.
   - Inform the nurse if any tasks such as charting have not been completed.
   - Leave the patient comfortable, turning him or her as necessary.

4. Other random thoughts
   - The staff is always grateful to those students who help answer call lights.
   - Students should listen closely when the doctor is in the room, as it is an opportunity to learn.

Essential Facts

- You are a guest; act like one. Positive relationships with the nursing staff are paramount.
- Staff nurses are ultimately responsible for the patients.

Reference

Goleman, D. (1995). *Emotional intelligence.* New York, NY: Bantam.

5

Organize the Semester—Have a Plan

Instructors are required to review the rules and requirements of the facility where they conduct each clinical rotation. The goal of this chapter is to provide blueprints for the first day of a clinical rotation. Each rotation can last from 4 days to 14 weeks, meeting once, twice, or three times a week. Because each instructor spends most of the first day preparing and reviewing printed or online expectations and guidelines for students, this chapter presents a template of an orientation day schedule. The sample guides and rules are adaptable to any setting. They have been developed by the authors and used by them quite effectively. A *bonus* is a valuable tool developed by a recent graduate. This gem is a template that includes all of the aspects that any student needs to know for change of shift report, vital assessment and care planning data, tips on working with a patient, and postconference tools.

In this chapter, you will learn:

- What to do before the first day with your students
- How to organize and conduct your first day with your clinical students
- Which blueprints can be most effectively used with the printed or online guidelines to enhance your students'

(continued)

orientation to the unit and their understanding of responsibilities
- The benefit of preparing and procuring a signed clinical expectation statement from the student after your orientation day

BEFORE THE FIRST DAY OF THE SEMESTER

Who are your students? Does the facility being used for the clinical rotation need their names in advance to facilitate their access to the site's computer system? What clinical experiences have they already had? Will they have concurrent classroom concentration on the specialty being taught at the clinical site? Some schools do not coordinate classroom and clinical topics, so your preparation needs to consider that. Is your clinical rotation considered a pass/fail course or will it result in an actual grade? If graded, you have a more challenging job. More than a few students are accustomed to receiving high grades and may not be pleased to learn that an "A" grade for a clinical rotation involves more than simply showing up on time. It is not unusual for the clinical site itself to augment the clinical instructor's planning with its own set of expectations. A sample appears in Exhibit 5.1.

Depending on the clinical site, you may need to spend at least 2 days by yourself on the new unit in advance of the rotation to get oriented. If you have been on a particular unit with students previously, it is still prudent to revisit for 4 to 6 hours if there has been a gap in time since your last experience there. Policies, procedures, equipment, staffing, and computer systems can change seemingly overnight, and you want to avoid the situation in which you are orienting your new students with inaccurate information. The benefit of time spent on the unit—ideally with two different nurses—cannot be overemphasized. Besides showing that you respect them and regard them as the true experts on their units, you will enhance your relationship with the staff, and their goodwill will likely extend to the students you bring on to the floor.

After your own orientation to the new unit, you can begin to develop your plan for the first day on the floor with your students. Think ahead! You must find a way to communicate to your students when and where you will meet on their first day. After all, the

Exhibit 5.1

Information List for Clinical Instructors

New clinical instructors are required to meet with the clinical nurse educator/patient care manager prior to the arrival of the students in order to:

1. Clarify patient assignments to ensure that they are appropriate for students.
2. Enhance communication and clinical planning with staff, manager, and educator.
3. Schedule time on the unit shadowing a staff nurse to become familiar with unit routines.
4. Complete a unit-specific agreement.
5. Submit other required paperwork:
    - An electronic spreadsheet with instructor and student names, along with other relevant information required by the site's security policy to procure computer system access
    - A statement of responsibility and confidentiality
    - Current curriculum vitae of the instructor
    - Clinical review form
6. Adhere to policy regarding student assignments:
    - Instructors are responsible for making student assignments.
    - Do not assign a student to a registered nurse who already has a staff orientee.
    - Inform staff about students who will be administering medications.
    - The supervisor must supervise all student medication administration.
    - All assessments must be done early, with related documentation signed by the instructor.
    - Ensure that your students are aware that no cell phone use is permitted on the units.

---

educational experience can be greatly diminished if they do not show up! Here are some possibilities for getting the word out:

- Ask the course coordinator to announce the time and place of the first meeting to your group at the facility, as well as to provide maps and directions online.
- Meet the group members at the school when they have class and provide the same information.
- Use the school's online learning management system to send an e-mail to provide the initial information.

The goal is to ensure that your clinical group clearly understands the place, time, and attire for the first clinical day. Be clear. Instead of saying, "Meet me in the lobby of the building," be specific. Say, instead, "Meet me in front of the big clock in the Smith lobby at 8 a.m. sharp!" Provide a map with written directions. Do not forget about nourishment. Often this is a 4- to 6-hour day, so inform the students about the lunch possibilities or dinner if you are supervising an evening clinical. Refer to Appendix A for further guidelines to assist you on orientation day.

ORGANIZE

Reserving Space

You must reserve space at the clinical site to conduct your orientation. Most hospitals have a limited number of conference rooms, so you may need to speak with the level coordinator. However, it is more likely that you, the clinical instructor, will have to obtain that information yourself, either from the nurse educator or the manager assigned to your clinical site.

Whether you will be instructing for 8 days or 8 weeks, *an organized and thorough orientation day will reap dividends* throughout the semester and promote a successful and enjoyable clinical experience for you, your students, and the patients and staff with whom you will be working.

Orientation Day

Have everything you expect of your students in a written form that they can keep for reference throughout the rotation. Often students will not remember all of the rules and expectations now facing them, and benefit from a written guide to fall back on. Design a schedule or calendar showing what is due and when (Exhibit 5.2). They will thank you later for it. It is also recommended that following your review of what is required of them, you have the students sign off on a brief statement saying "I have read and had an opportunity to ask questions about the expectations for [course name and number]." This step will mitigate the potential for problems down the road that students would otherwise blame on uncertainty or confusion relating to their course responsibilities.

Let us pause here to add a word about the second-career (or second-degree) students introduced in Chapter 3; they especially appreciate notice of all course expectations as soon as possible! They are likely running their own households as well as coordinating child care, parent care, and job demands that are competing for their attention at the

Exhibit 5.2

Sample Schedule of Due Dates

1	Monday	Jan 11	First day clinical orientation lecture at _____, Mental Status Exam (MSE video)
			Meet briefly; please review all of the paperwork that I give you and jot down questions to be answered at the Veterans Administration on Jan 13. BRING ALL PAPERWORK I GIVE YOU ON Jan 13.
2	Wednesday	Jan 13	Bring envelopes with all the information that I gave you and we will review each paper one by one. Security clearance needs two forms of ID. *BRING THIS SCHEDULE DAILY.*
			Meet at 7:30 a.m. in lobby with Starbucks station (please read paperwork I gave you on Monday with questions documented). *BRING LUNCH!!!*
			CASE STUDY ASSIGNMENT WILL BE DISTRIBUTED.
3	Monday		No clinical rotation (Martin Luther King Day)
4	Wednesday	Jan 20	Meet in room 9 of the lab area.
			Clinical Standardized Patient (SP) experience MSE/Lab MSE Prep Sheet and Hearing Voices That Are Distressing (HVTAD) Simulation (at Villanova 7:45 a.m.–2:00 p.m.) wear uniform. Complete paperwork described by Dr. Bradley in N 3120.

CALENDAR CONTINUES...

same time they are handling their clinical rotation with its attendant work. In their efforts to manage their often complicated lives, second-career students are eager to know what you will require of them even if your related communication reaches them before the rotation actually starts.

Tell your students to write their nonurgent questions down during the course of the clinical day. Allowing them to do this anonymously will avoid any embarrassment they might feel in asking about something that they believe everyone else already knows.

Ask Each Student to Define His or Her Goals for the Clinical Practicum Rotation

Collect this information from your students. Give each student a copy of his or her response, and keep one for yourself. If you have this information early in the day, you can better gauge and redefine student expectations. The level coordinator may have given you objectives and goals, but the students may have completely different ideas. If such a discrepancy exists, you need to adjust your orientation by better educating students about the school and the coordinator's objectives. Flexibility is paramount in this role.

Confirm Their Mathematical Competency

If students are administering medications in the clinical practicum, it is prudent to give them a brief and simple medication calculation quiz that requires knowledge of basic math, such as ratio and proportion, and intravenous drip rate equations. Students should be reminded that almost every new registered nurse in a health care facility must pass a medication calculation quiz as a condition of hire. Be sure to acquaint the students with the basic abbreviations used by the institution for the protection of you and the patients. For example, QID means four times a day, but you should specify what four times your institution designates as appropriate, for example, 8 a.m., 12 p.m., 4 p.m., and 8 p.m. This cursory evaluation allows you to see if some students need to be sent back to the learning lab for review before they are allowed to administer medications.

Establish the Course Requirements

Like students everywhere, your charges want to know the "bottom line." What do they have to do to pass this clinical rotation? It is a key question, and you should not hesitate to address it. Each clinical instructor brings his or her personality and style to the instruction. The students need to know what you judge as important for their success. Clinical rotations may be pass/fail or result in a letter or numeric grade. All students need a copy of the school's clinical evaluation tool at the outset of the clinical experience, and you should review each line or item with them. Part IV reviews the types of grading systems available in many nursing programs. Exhibit 5.3 presents one such grading guide, which reflects actual examples of students with whom Professor Stabler-Haas has previously worked.

Exhibit 5.3

Grading Guide for Competency Evaluation Instrument (CEI)

NUR 3121 (Psych) **Prof. Stabler-Haas**

The CEI is composed of 10 distinct objectives (worth 70% of the final grade) as well as a case study paper (worth 30% of the final grade). This allows you to formulate a realistic expectation regarding grading for this course's 10 objectives.

Grade	Explanation	Examples of student performance
4	The superlative level of performance associated with this grade makes it challenging to obtain.	Presented at least twice to patient groups Exceeded expectation in written assignments—received a 4 in interactional goal sheet (follows sample provided closely), community paper, medication presentation (presentation and handouts to peers), etc. Correlated clinical and theory in peer conferences consistently Researched at least two topics that group benefited from and presented them Implemented above criteria nursing care to a patient (e.g., initiated contact with a social worker for a patient who required new glasses) Discussed patient medication at every postconference Earned an "A" on case study paper, which is necessary to receive a 4 in certain criteria reflected in case study *Was truly present with patients* Initiated teaching to staff or patients: nursing care to patients such as vital signs and helping with hygiene or wound care with nurse Consistently asked staff what to do to help Correlated *mind/body information* such as patient is on antihypertensive that increases risk of depression or patient's family are abusive and the patient now is violent

(continued)

Exhibit 5.3

Grading Guide for Competency Evaluation Instrument (CEI) (*continued*)

Grade	Explanation	Examples of student performance
3	This level of performance represents an above-average demonstration of clinical skills.	Presented one group to patients Exceeded expectation in most written work (achieved 3s) Researched at least one topic and presented to group Earned a "B" on case study paper, which is necessary to receive 3 in certain criteria reflected in case study Initiated teaching to staff or patients: nursing care to patients such as vital signs; teaching about medications, etc.; and assisting nurse with wound care or hygiene needs of patients Asked staff what to do to help *Was truly present with patients* Correlated *mind/body information* such as patient is on antihypertensive that increases risk of depression or patient's family are abusive and the patient now is violent
2	This level of performance meets—but does not exceed—expectations as they relate to clinical performance. According to past marking history, a 2 has been assigned 10% of the time.	Did not present to group Met expectations in written assignments Rarely correlated theory to clinical and did no additional research Prepared case study paper that just met criteria
1	This level of performance demonstrates a lack of the basic skills expected at the clinical site, and constitutes failure of the objective. A 1 in any objective prevents the student from passing the course.	Absent and did not call instructor before 6:30 that morning Was late for clinical rotation Used uncivil behavior to peers, staff, or patients Used inappropriate language to peers, patients, staff, or instructor

Exhibit 5.3

Grading Guide for Competency Evaluation Instrument (CEI) (*continued*)

Grade	Explanation	Examples of student performance
		Sat in back of room and did not interact with patients
		Fell asleep during clinical rotation
		Used cell phone during part of clinical day, including waiting for preconferences and postconferences
		Did not participate in preconferences or postconferences
		Does not submit assignments in a timely manner and/or missed assignments or needed to be reminded individually by professor about due assignments

Being on time and present each day is always an expectation for performance and contributes to your ability to exceed criteria.

- You may think that I do not observe you in clinical rotation as much as the instructor did in medical–surgical nursing. I am observing from a distance and always check quietly with staff weekly about all students and their interactions. This is a different type of observation than I do when I teach med–surg in the summer with all of you.
- Again, the case study paper due at the end of the rotation is worth 30% of your grade, as mentioned in all classes. We will discuss expectations for the paper at the outset of the course and meet one on one at a later point (outline day) as described in the calendar of clinical assignments that I gave you prior to the beginning of the rotation to examine your case study outline.
- Students who have received 3 and 4 in the competencies in the past put much time into the case study outline that is due weeks earlier by using the *Suggestions for Case Study* paper in the N 3121 Blackboard syllabus that Dr. Bradley provided. The more questions and time that you put into this outline and paper, the more it reflects in your grade.
- I welcome your questions and can meet with any student any day at clinical. I am a part-time faculty member and on campus infrequently, but you have my cell number and you can call me with questions as well as e-mail me.

Thank you,
Prof. Stabler-Haas

Remember, it is your goal to foster independence and safety in each student's clinical experience. Do not hesitate to expect students to arrive early on clinical units to begin their preparation for the day's responsibilities. You do not need to do all of the prep work. Students can arrive early (6:15 a.m.) and talk with the night nurses about patient assignments and gather needed information to present to you in your preconference at 7 a.m. As long as it is established that they cannot go into patient rooms without your presence on the unit and that they are respectful of the nurses' time constraints, this opportunity can foster mutual teaching, connection, and responsibility in your developing nursing students.

Key Components

The following key components must be included in your verbal presentation and in any handouts to students on Day 1, your orientation day.

- The clinical hours that are required. For example, hours are Tuesdays and Thursdays from 7 a.m. to 1 p.m. and Wednesdays from 6:30 a.m. to 6:30 p.m.
- The required dates of the clinical rotation. Include any school events or holidays on which there are no clinical days. Establish lines of communication between you and your students and among the students themselves in the event of school closure, and so forth. Will you text, e-mail, call, have a phone chain? You must address this issue on Day 1.
- The essential expectations that you and the nursing program manager deem most important. For example, attendance and punctuality may be the most basic criteria for assessing performance. If students are not present or not on time, it is difficult to assess performance. Remind them this is all part of their professionalism.
- Be specific in communicating the attendance policy. Contact information should be provided. If the student will be late or absent, how and when do you require him or her to notify you and the unit? If the student needs to contact you at other times during the week, tell him or her the best way, either by e-mail, text, or phone. In discussing how missed days are to be handled, avoid the use of the term "make-up" unless your school actually adds a day to the calendar for this purpose. In terms of make-up submissions, there is simply no offsite paperwork that can replace the treasure

trove of experience that is packed into a student's clinical day. Yet, in many students' minds, if they do make-up work as a result of an absence, it is as if they did not miss the clinical day. So instead, use the words "alternate assignment" in describing outside work that will meet the course objectives but can never provide the richness of learning by immersion that is available only at the clinical site. See Chapter 16 for more information on alternate assignments.

- Give sample documentation flow sheets to the students. The Student Report Sheet in Appendix D is a wonderful tool developed by Rachel Yoder when she was a nursing student. It provides forms your students can use to write their assessments and notes. If your institution uses electronic charting, first familiarize yourself with this system and then adapt it to your students' needs. Many institutions require that you and your students have completed multiple training modules online to prepare for your role in their institution. Often, written evidence of completing these essential modules is required to be given to the manager or nurse educator on or before Day 1. Your course coordinator or program coordinator will provide further direction as they will have already heard from the hospitals. Find out if each student can receive a password to gain entry into the documentation system as soon as possible—the students will need practice with this skill.
- Journals may also be required. See Appendix B for an instructor's template of written journal requirements.
- Tell your students your policy concerning future written letters of reference (see Chapter 20).
- Prepare and procure a signed clinical expectation statement after your orientation day (Exhibit 5.4).

Exhibit 5.4

Clinical Expectations Signature Sheet

[Instructor name] Clinical Rotation for NSL 311

I have read [instructor name] guidelines for clinical expectations for ABC Hospital. I have had the opportunity to ask questions about the expectations and I understand the expectations.

_____ (signature)
_____ (date)
Distributed November 1, 20XX

Students' eyes may start to glaze over after about 1 hour of clinical orientation. No matter how interesting and important your information may be, students will gradually lose interest in your "pearls of wisdom." By mentioning that they will need to sign the document shown in Exhibit 5.4 at the end of the day, even the most reserved and quiet students immediately discover questions that they urgently need answered. The signed document may also assist you later in the rotation when and if a student asserts that you never told him or her "not to give medications without you." If you have your guidelines and instructions in writing and keep a copy with the student's signed signature sheet, you will have a more successful outcome counseling a student who failed to heed your orientation instructions.

Emphasize the Students' Responsibilities While in the Unit

The nurses in your unit must be confident that your students will properly discharge all their responsibilities before you all leave the unit. For example, if you agree to have the students document a full assessment, perform hygiene care, and administer medications, you must ensure that these tasks are completed before you and the students end the clinical day. If they are not done, the staff will become distrustful and disinclined to allow you or your students to care for their patients. They may also hesitate to teach and share knowledge with your students. One fact cannot be overemphasized—*the instructor's relationships with the staff and nurse unit manager are paramount for a successful clinical experience* for the students and for the instructor. Post a written guide to the staff of the student's responsibilities while on the unit.

Take the Tour

At the beginning or end of orientation day, the instructor may schedule a visit to the unit. If you arrange this visit at the end of the day, remember that students may have already reached their saturation point for absorbing information. The middle of the day is best because the unit is a little less frantic, you have not yet exhausted their attention span, and they may welcome a new activity at that point. You may only be able to give them a handout with essential codes to use to gain entry into kitchens, utility rooms, and medication rooms. The handout can include a sample schedule of their clinical day or a list of their patients (see Appendix C for a sample student schedule). Another suggestion is to let the students review a patient chart and have them walk around and tour the unit on their own. Many nursing instructors distribute a "scavenger hunt" guide (see Exhibit 5.5) for the students to use during their initial orientation tour on the unit.

Exhibit 5.5

Scavenger Hunt for XYZ Skilled Nursing Facility

Please find the following items. If the hunt involves a person, note the name and any information that might be helpful for our group. If it is a thing, jot down where you found it. We will discuss your results at postconference today.

1. Clean linens to change a bed
2. The nurse in charge and two other nurses (introduce yourself)
3. Kitchen supplies
4. Medication, IV room, and Pyxis
5. The residents' personal toothpaste, deodorant, soap, and so forth
6. Residents' charts and computers accessible by students
7. The latest record of patients' medications
8. The nurse who is caring for your patient (remember your own introduction—name and school)
9. The nurse's assistant who is caring for your patient (remember your own introduction)
10. Location of thermometer, pulse oximeter, blood pressure measurement device
11. Unit secretary (remember your own introduction)
12. Electronic system to find vital patient information

This is a good start. Feel free to record anything else that you learned and all questions noted as you complete this sheet.

Essential Facts

- Begin by learning clinical site expectations before you even meet your students.
- Be organized and have a plan for orientation day. A well-executed orientation day will pay many dividends.
- Provide detailed written information and distribute a copy to students.
- Ensure that all student responsibilities are completed before leaving the unit each day

6

Confidentiality and Patient Privacy

Use discretion always. In other words, do not talk about patients in the elevators, in public spaces, or in front of individuals not specifically designated by the patient to receive information. This chapter provides specific examples of students who violated patient privacy by speaking "innocently" about their patients outside of the clinical setting. Information will be given about maintaining patient privacy while delivering care in the unit.

In this chapter, you will learn:

- Relevant provisions of the Health Insurance Portability and Accountability Act (HIPAA) and how it interfaces with your students
- Ways in which students can violate patient privacy
- Basic suggestions to avoid violations of privacy

CONCEPTS OF CONFIDENTIALITY AND PATIENT PRIVACY

Maintaining the confidentiality of patient health care information is both a legislative and professional imperative, as underscored by the Health Insurance Portability and Accountability Act (HIPAA) of 1996 and the American Nurses Association (ANA, 2015) *Code of Ethics*. HIPAA was designed to increase the confidentiality of patient information.

Students may be on the same units as their neighbors, peers, or family and friends. It cannot be emphasized enough that absolutely *no* information about any patient can be discussed with anyone outside of the unit's perimeter. When a breach occurs, litigation can follow.

Applying HIPAA to the Clinical Setting

Most nursing programs teach the concepts of patient privacy and confidentiality in the classroom as part of their Nursing Fundamentals course, because it is considered "essential" knowledge prior to beginning any clinical practicum rotation. Your students may have been informed about HIPAA and the legal implications of not protecting patient information, but the actual practice of enforcing patient privacy in the clinical field is another matter. As a nursing instructor, you must educate your students and monitor their discussions to ensure that the privacy of each patient is protected. Never hesitate to impress upon these future practicing nurses how this is a vital function of their role and a nursing duty as highlighted in the ANA's *Code of Ethics* (ANA, 2015).

Visitors and Family Members

The goal is to apply HIPAA content to the clinical practicum. The clinical instructor must ascertain the degree of student understanding of patient privacy and confidentiality. Most importantly, the clinical instructor needs to relate HIPAA requirements to the clinical setting. In an acute care setting, for example, there are multiple times when students may encounter visitors at their patients' bedsides. They have to be careful to whom they speak and what information they convey to these visitors. There have been occasions on which visiting family and neighbors received health information that they should not have been given.

Another potential problem involves the specific information you may share with the patient's family members. It is the patient—not the health care provider—who controls the disclosure of health information. You must *obtain the patient's permission* before you can discuss his or her medical condition with the family. If family members are present in the room and the patient asks you questions, you are still on somewhat shaky ground. It is prudent to discuss with patients beforehand what information they want discussed and shared with family members. If you have any doubts, ask the family to briefly leave the room and then ask the patient to clarify what areas are acceptable to discuss. You can also ask the patient to sign a consent form before the discussion takes place, especially if sensitive material is to be discussed. Information about AIDS, sexually transmitted diseases, substance abuse, and psychiatric illness is considered especially sensitive.

Social Media

Student nurses do not fully grasp who they are speaking to and how the HIPAA regulations apply to all conversations in the patient care setting. Students are too overwhelmed with the duties imposed by their instructors and the overall task of navigating the complexities of the clinical environment. Sometimes, just looking for equipment in order to obtain vital signs is a big stressor. Students are not in the clinical learning environment on a daily basis, so when they do drop in for their practicum rotations, they are constantly adjusting to the changes they see and experience. As a result, protecting patient health information may not be their immediate concern.

Clinical instructors need to continue to be on top of this and continue to enforce patient privacy. What may also compound the situation is assistance received from staff nurses. These nurses are more than willing to help students and may inadvertently share lab work or other patient information that was printed out from the hospital computer. This act of sharing paperwork (with patient information) is another risk factor for potential HIPAA violations. Commonly, students inadvertently take this paperwork home.

Students have problems grasping the realities of confidentiality. That is why inadvertent or unintentional breaches of confidentiality occur and will continue to occur. Advances in social media and technology have contributed to confidentiality breaches. Because of this, some clinical site agencies have banned the use of any kind of phone on their floors to prevent these problems. Nursing programs have established policies on the use of social media. This can be found in most student handbooks. It has to be stressed to students and health care workers alike that postings on social media can result in civil liability to patients, job loss, disciplinary action by state boards of nursing, and criminal investigations (Hader & Brown, 2010). According to Melnik (2013), the Health Information Technology for Economic and Clinical Health (HITECH) Act has stronger privacy and security protections of patient data. Melnik's article clearly identifies nursing regulations as well as federal and state laws addressing patient health information. More importantly she depicts the various legal consequences for nurses and health care workers. Melnik provides a nice reminder for all of us, "when in doubt, *do not* submit" (p. 8).

Exposure to real-life cases or case scenarios depicting violations of confidentiality and privacy may help students understand this important issue. The National Council of State Boards of Nursing (NCSBN) has a nice pamphlet on the use of social media, which is readily accessible (www.ncsbn.org/NCSBN_SocialMedia.pdf). In addition, the NCSBN has an educational video showing what can happen when a nurse takes a picture of a beloved patient and posts the picture and comments online (NCSBN Regulatory Innovations Department, 2011). The ANA also has several resources for nurses and students; one such resource is a toolkit (ANA, n.d.). The case studies in this chapter further illustrate the need for students to uphold privacy. Clinical instructors may read these or share with their students prior to the start of their clinical rotation time.

CASE STUDIES

The case studies in Exhibits 6.1 and 6.2 present two different scenarios that emphasize the need for each instructor to stress daily to students that *patient confidentiality is paramount.*

As these cases demonstrate, the aphorism that encourages the "ounce of prevention" rings especially true in the clinical setting. One must also emphasize the need for privacy while on the unit itself. This

Exhibit 6.1

Hannah's Scenario

During Hannah's geriatric rotation, she cared for an 80-year-old patient. She did an excellent job and was complimented by her instructor and by the staff. She went home and told her family how much she enjoyed caring for this patient and what happened during her day. She mentioned the patient's name to her family, thinking that he lived in a different town and that no one could possibly know him. Based on the circumstances of the patient's case, the student's mother correctly concluded that the patient was in fact the father of one of her employees. This worker had missed a lot of time lately supposedly because of personal illness. She became angry that her employee was not ill as she had claimed, but rather was taking time off to be with her father. The student was very concerned that her mother would reprimand the staff member, causing the employee to subsequently question how the mother had obtained this information. The student now wondered if she needed to inform her nursing instructor of the confidentiality breach.

Exhibit 6.2

Grace's Scenario

Grace had to present her patient to her clinical group and was preparing the presentation in her dormitory room. She had her patient's name on all of the information that she was preparing and left the presentation material on her desk. Later in the day, her former high school friends came to visit and planned to stay overnight in her room. One friend read the information on her desk and exclaimed that the patient was her boyfriend's mother. She also said that her boyfriend does not live with his mother and was not aware of his mother's clinical psychiatric situation. She began to call him on her cell phone to inform him that his mom was in a psychiatric facility. Grace pleaded with her to not call and tried to explain how she would be in serious trouble if this information about the patient was revealed.

---

means that all computer screens must be turned off when students are not using them. If a visitor simply walks past an unattended computer screen and inadvertently sees patient information, a violation of privacy has occurred and liability could possibly result for those nurses on the unit.

Essential Facts

- Teach students the important elements concerning patient privacy and health information.
- No information should be divulged without consent.
- Before sharing information with families, confer with patients.

References

American Nurses Association. (n.d.). Social networking principles toolkit. Retrieved from http://nursingworld.org/socialnetworkingtoolkit.aspx

American Nurses Association. (2015). *Code of ethics for nurses with interpretive statements.* Silver Spring, MD: Nursesbooks.org. Retrieved from www.nursingworld.org/MainMenuCategories/EthicsStandards/Codeof EthicsforNurses/Code-of-Ethics-For-Nurses.html

Hader, A. L., & Brown, E. D. (2010). Patient privacy in social media. *American Association of Nurse Anesthetists Journal, 78*(4), 269–274.

Melnik, T. (2013). Avoiding violations of patient privacy with social media. *Missouri State Board of Nursing Newsletter, 15*(3), 7–10.

NCSBN Regulatory Innovations Department. (2011). *Social media guidelines for nurses* [Video file]. Retrieved from https://www.ncsbn.org/347.htm

III

Getting to Know Your Nursing Students: Who Are the Best and Who Are the Rest?

7

The High Fliers: How to Screen for Higher Achieving Students

One of the challenging aspects of clinical teaching is managing students during the limited blocks of time available for instructor observation. Practicing nurses work 8- or 12-hour shifts, whereas student nurses are usually at the clinical sites for 4- to 8-hour blocks of time. As a result, many clinical instructors try to see things "early." That is, most seasoned clinical instructors try to identify or classify their students within the first week of the clinical rotation. One such classification would be students "at risk" (at risk of failing the course) and students "not at risk."

In this chapter, you will learn:

- The characteristics of students who are not at risk, those who are considered "high fliers"
- The advantages of classifying students early in the program

ASSESSING STUDENT CAPABILITIES

The clinical instructor is first and foremost a teacher. To become an effective teacher, the instructor must assist students to learn to problem solve and think at a higher level. Therefore, the successful instructor needs to develop quick insight into the nature and capabilities of the students. Within the first 2 weeks of the clinical rotation, the instructor should be able to distinguish between the *high fliers*, those who will potentially receive higher grades, and the *not-so-high fliers*, whose success cannot be immediately ensured.

IDENTIFYING THE HIGH FLIERS

This distinction is also important because the clinical instructor faces certain stresses when dealing with a student who is at risk of failing the clinical course. The first sign of possible failure is unsatisfactory behavior when performing a nursing skill. The instructor needs to take extra time to manage this behavior while continuing to teach the other students within the time frame set by the nursing program.

Surprisingly, for some instructors, identifying the high fliers is quite easy. Some use instinct. For example, some students may impress you by completing homework earlier than the rest of the group or by earning a high grade on the medication quiz. Sometimes, a student's question may give you an impression of that student's cognitive ability. For example, one student may ask, "I just took vitals on my patient. What do I do next?" In comparison, another student may voice, "I took vitals on my patient. Now I am starting the nursing assessment because I plan to give the medications soon." Obviously, the second student has a clear understanding of the nursing process and can initiate interventions competently. Initiating interventions competently is a major objective for student nurses, because it is a basic requirement and goal of graduation. This goal, as well as other goals for students, is usually documented in the student handbook of most nursing programs.

CHARACTERISTICS OF HIGH FLIERS

Based on years of experience and bearing witness to all kinds of student behaviors, the following are the most common characteristics of high fliers.

1. *The student is prepared each clinical day and displays this during the clinical rotation.*

    This student has reviewed his or her patient assignment and has some knowledge base to share with you about the patient's condition. If assigned to give medications that day, he or she will have medications reviewed and written down. This student may even present you with pages of written or typed notes of the work he or she did in preparing for the clinical day. Those papers will include information about the patient's medical disease process and the management of the medications. Each medication the patient is prescribed may be documented. The student will also bring his or her own books to the clinical facility.

2. *The student communicates well orally with you and the patients.*

    This student asks you questions about the patient and can clearly verbalize some information about the assigned patient. When observed, this student is comfortable at the bedside speaking to the patient and the staff nurses. The student may show initiative by, for example, showing you various online resources retrieved from an Internet search.

3. *The student prioritizes patient interventions appropriately.*

    For example, in a medical–surgical dayshift rotation, without your direction you witness the student rechecking a heart rate because the patient complained of dizziness. Another example is, at a community rotation, the student may check the vital signs and promptly report to you or the staff nurse an abnormal blood pressure and heart rate. This student may even ask a staff nurse to recheck the vital signs with him or her for accuracy.

REFLECTION JOURNALS WRITTEN BY HIGH FLIERS

Reflection or student journals are an example of written work where students may also reveal their goals and reflect on their past experiences. Students write about the clinical experiences that they want to share with their instructor. At many schools, this is an ongoing assignment due at the end of each week. In these journals, high fliers may impress you with what they have written. Many times, what they write shows you the high level of thinking they have applied to their experiences with patients or in the thought processes they have displayed with certain skills. In addition, these journals serve as a communication path for student and teacher. You will get to know the cognitive and behavioral aspects of each student. High fliers are usually solid writers who provide more detail and self-evaluation of their work. At times, they may be more critical or have more goals for themselves. Journals are just one example of written work that can reveal many aspects of your students.

Essential Facts

- It is best to distinguish the high fliers early.
- High fliers are prepared, communicate at a higher level, and can prioritize nursing interventions better.

8

The Not-So-High Fliers: How to Screen for Potential "Problem Students"

Teaching in the clinical setting requires an enormous amount of preparation before the course begins and then prior to each clinical day. One major frustration for instructors is the limited time available at the clinical site to teach all the students. In some acute care settings, the student-to-instructor ratio is a surprising 10:1. State boards of nursing are well aware of this fact. One practice that can assist the clinical instructor is the early identification of strong students (high fliers) and weak students (not-so-high fliers). Often, you as the instructor can strategize ways for the high fliers to assist and provide needed role modeling for the not-so-high fliers.

In this chapter, you will learn:

- The characteristics of the not-so-high fliers
- How to compare high fliers and not-so-high fliers
- Strategies to assist the not-so-high fliers

IDENTIFYING AT-RISK STUDENTS

Instructors need to "see it early," according to Teeter (2001). That is, they need to identify the at-risk students or the not-so-high fliers by certain "red flags." Some of these red flags are: "The student arrives late on the first or second day" or the student is "unengaged with learning" or the student "frequently gets staff and other students to help" (Teeter, 2001, p. 91). Sometimes, you may at first think that some students have really good relationships with the staff of nurses, nurse assistants, and technicians, particularly as you witness their close interactions. But this can be a warning sign. It is wise to keep an extra careful eye on these students just to make sure that they are doing their work and not just "copying" data from what has already been documented. They could even be getting answers to your questions from the staff nurses!

"Seeing it early" is a good strategy to use as a clinical instructor. The not-so-high fliers may be more difficult to notice. Develop a keen sense of awareness. For example, some instructors might automatically stigmatize students who stay at the patient's bedside or are difficult to find during the clinical day. However, these students may not be at risk. Yes, it is true that students who are nowhere to be found may be "hiding" from you and your questions about their patients' care, but those students may also just be spending time caring for their assigned patients and being extremely attentive to the needs of those patients. You need to discern these differences.

CHARACTERISTICS OF NOT-SO-HIGH FLIERS

A few characteristics of the not-so-high fliers and a discussion of each are listed in Table 8.1.

Table 8.1

High Fliers Versus Not-So-High Fliers	
High Flier	**Not-So-High Flier**
1. Prepares for each clinical day	1. Does not thoroughly prepare for the clinical day
2. Communicates clearly with instructor and/or patients and staff nurses	2. Is inconsistent with communication (e.g., may not have verbalized to you an abnormal vital sign)
3. Prioritizes patient interventions appropriately	3. Is unsure about patient care priorities

1. *The student is not thoroughly prepared each clinical day.*

    In most cases, there is a great deal of self-directed preparation on behalf of the student. Not-so-high fliers, however, will be unprepared even though they may have been instructed to prepare for a particular procedure, such as Foley catheter insertion or medication shot. Another example is assigned written work. Whatever the case, the not-so-high fliers will not turn in their work or will turn in work that is incomplete.

    Whether the assignment is written or oral, the not-so-high fliers will have an excuse as to why their performance is not up to par and why they are "unprepared." More often than not, the clinical instructor will witness such a student sitting in the back of a nursing lounge with an open textbook, writing down the information that he or she should have arrived with at the beginning of the clinical day. This student may also be observed in clandestine discussion with more prepared fellow students in an apparent attempt to obtain answers to questions that you have previously posed to this not-so-high flier.

2. *The student is inconsistent in communicating information (e.g., the student may not have informed you of a patient with a high blood pressure [BP] value).*

    The not-so-high fliers are less assertive than the others in the group. That is, they are more comfortable being spoken to than actually initiating a conversation with you! As a result, they may not convey information promptly. They may know they are hearing something abnormal in the lungs or note a higher BP value in a patient, but they cannot decide what the next step should be. They do not speak to the staff nurse or a fellow student to seek feedback. In fact, instead of speaking to anyone about their suspicions, they keep the information to themselves.

    The instructor should allow for the possibility that inadequate communication may be the result of inherent shyness and not a lack of knowledge or preparation. Therefore, the instructor must do some careful probing before judging the student's potential. Although students who are shy may avoid eye contact or nonverbal behavior, this does not necessarily mean they are not-so-high fliers. Further questioning of the student in a private place or in your office may be warranted to gain a bit more understanding of the student. Taking away part of the anxiety (being in the role of a clinical student during a clinical performance day) may actually help you get more insight into your student.

3. *The student is unsure about patient care priorities.*

    The not-so-high fliers struggle with prioritizing basic care for their patients. To them, every intervention is a priority. A morning bath may be more important than getting the morning vital signs. Providing the evening snack as soon as it arrives may be more important than checking if the patient is diabetic and needs insulin first. They may not know that assessment of heart sounds is a priority action before administering a prescribed beta blocker medication. This problem with prioritization may either be a thinking problem or a problem related to self-induced anxiety. For example, a patient may have just woken up and asked the student to set up a bath. Not thinking through the care tasks for the day, the student happily helps the patient get this done before all other assessments.

    Every clinical rotation has expectations of basic student competencies and skills. It is expected that students advance through each rotation and make improvements within a given clinical rotation. This is most true in medical–surgical settings where nurses care for multiple patients with various medical needs. Nurses are taught to prioritize their actions. They learn this skill during clinical rotations with clinical instructors. This is also true in community health rotations where students may not always be working in close proximity to their clinical instructors. In these rotations, students have to be more diligent to understand their work-related goals and priorities. They may conduct a health screening and not be able to prioritize the problems revealed during the screening.

MONITORING THE NOT-SO-HIGH FLIERS

Once you have some idea of which students are the not-so-high fliers in your clinical group, keep a critical eye on them. That's it! It is also wise to be attuned to comments from staff nurses about these students. If these students are not performing their required duties, you will hear about this from the nursing staff (especially if you have developed a collegial relationship with them). As noted in Chapter 4, students and the clinical instructor are guests in the unit. Thus, any tasks not completed by the student will be reported by the staff personnel to the nurse manager, who will then immediately notify you. Many instructors are not happy receiving a phone call about a missed task. Therefore, communicate clearly and early with your students about their responsibilities.

Another word of caution about the not-so-high fliers: They may also be those students who are habitually late in leaving the clinical site. That is, at the end of the clinical day, students usually gather at one spot to walk to their conference site for postconference, or they independently meet at a designated time and location for postconference. The at-risk student may lag behind one day and then the next and then the next. When it happens once, try to get the cause for the lateness—maybe a patient had an unexpected test or, for a home visit, maybe the patient was unavailable. If it happens repeatedly, it is a cause for concern. A similar finding for this student is that he or she may be the one that other students gather around. This may just be a casual student gathering, but this can also mean that the not-so-high flier has asked for and is receiving assistance from peers in answering questions.

One strategy that has great benefits for both high fliers and not-so-high fliers is pairing one student from each category and giving specific guidelines for this intervention. You can make this part of your total clinical experience and expectation for your rotation. For example, select one student from each flier category who will then collaborate as a two-person team. Of course, you will avoid any mention of your categories or your reasoning for the pairing. Have them work together to provide care for a group (two to four) of patients. One student will be the "professional nurse" and the other the nurse's patient care tech. It is the responsibility of the nurse to gather all information, communicate this to his or her team, procure or provide all needed care and information to the patients, communicate to the primary nurse, and do all of the reporting and documentation. These two roles should be reversed on the next clinical day with the same two students. Have the high flyer be the professional nurse on Day 1 of the experience, and the not-so-high flier assume the same responsibility on Day 2.

Here is the reaction of one student who participated in this role-sharing clinical experience:

> It was my first time pairing up with a partner and to experience team work, management, and delegation. Through this experience I once again learned about the crucial aspect of communication within a team. I was really grateful that I had the chance to work with another peer because it allowed me to delegate roles such as obtaining vital signs and communicating,

which was crucial because my patients were on meds that required taking a blood pressure or a pulse.

Do not forget to explain the aforementioned strategy to the staff on the unit ahead of time so they are aware of which student is responsible for each patient's needs.

Lastly, one of the most useful tools or strategies any clinical instructor can utilize is to coassign the student with a "willing" staff nurse. Basically, you first need to establish your collegial relationship with the staff, and then discuss the possibility of having your students (one by one) work alongside a primary nurse for the shift. Develop goals and objectives of the experience for the students to document along with their feelings and thoughts at the completion of the shift. The following are some comments from senior students after they spent a shift with a primary staff nurse:

> I really learned a lot from Kerry. It was amazing to see how good of a nurse she was, and how much she learned along the way just from practicing. It made me feel a bit more comfortable about the process of graduating and starting my experience as a real nurse. She taught me a lot of time-management skills, precision, detail-oriented skills, and how to accomplish everything you want to during a shift in a concise manner.

> Following Edie was such a great learning experience. It made me a little bit stressed out about all of the responsibilities of a nurse. I realized how organized I will have to be, and how important each and every task is, and how essential it is to be aware and present while you are working. These are not new ideas to me but this shadowing experience made it all that much more real. It also made me very excited to graduate and be independent!

If you need extra help monitoring some of the students, ask the staff. Seeking the staff's input is always a wise move, as it may or may not validate the traits that you see in the student. More frequently, though, the staff will come and inform you who they think are your higher level students. Unsolicited feedback about your students is a normal aspect of the clinical teaching arena.

To summarize, if you spot a not-so-high flier in your clinical group, just keep an eye on that student! No further action is needed on your part. You will be too busy with the normal day's tasks to do anything else with this student unless, of course, a problem occurs. The instructor may continue to observe unsatisfactory behavior. If you are seeing more "red flags" and are unsure about them, review Chapter 11. If more than one "flag" is identified, the instructor is now warned that the student is in jeopardy of clinical course failure. A more elaborate listing of these behaviors is given in Chapter 11.

Essential Facts

- Not-so-high fliers may be difficult to spot.
- High fliers can sometimes augment your own efforts in helping the not-so-high fliers improve their performance.
- Be open to the staff's input regarding certain students.

Reference

Teeter, M. (2001). Formula for success: Addressing unsatisfactory clinical performance. *Nurse Educator, 30*(3), 91–92.

IV

The Performance Appraisals: Clinical Evaluations

9

The Clinical Evaluation Triad

Most programs require that the student perform a self-evaluation of clinical performance, followed by the instructor's own evaluation of the student, along with the student's evaluation of the clinical instructor. Together, these three assessments form the clinical evaluation triad.

In this chapter, you will learn:

- The nature and purpose of each component of the clinical evaluation triad
- Suggestions for the instructor to use in guiding students toward a realistic evaluation
- A compassionate attitude to reviewing and incorporating students' evaluation of the instructor

STUDENT SELF-EVALUATION

Regardless of what type of evaluation tool is used, most nursing programs require students to perform a self-evaluation—two, actually, one at the middle of the course and one at the end. Usually, students submit their self-appraisals a few days before planned evaluations from the instructor. Included in both may be a written summary of strengths that the students feel they have and areas where they need to do work in the future. As their evaluator, you are teaching the students to accept and assume responsibility for their learning and performance. Meet with them individually, and emphasize that the value to be derived from the clinical experience is largely a product of their own efforts. The more initiative they invest in achieving an understanding of the nature of their patients' illnesses and the corresponding treatment modalities prescribed, the sturdier will be the conceptual foundation that they will soon carry into the work world.

These evaluations provide the nursing instructor with a blueprint to use in communicating expectations to students, who in turn will be better prepared to accurately assess their own performance. The midterm student self-evaluation is a particularly useful tool, in that it illuminates performance issues that there is still time to resolve. Students are required to rate their own performance based on the objectives set by the program and the clinical instructor, so they may initially need assistance in understanding how to effectively complete their very first self-evaluation. Take the opportunity to add your comments and specific instructions to the student self-evaluation and state how a student can improve performance.

According to Gaberson and Oermann (2010), development of self-evaluation skills is paramount for nurses. Because nurses must be competent in a practice that involves daily management of patients' illnesses and the skillful use of pharmacological therapies and lifesaving equipment, it is essential that nurses continuously self-monitor their performances. Throughout their careers, nurses must determine when they need more education or skill training. It is important, therefore, to foster the development of self-evaluation skill in the student nurse. Exhibit 9.1 is an example of a student self-evaluation.

Although many students report that the process of self-evaluation can provoke anxiety, their preliminary discomfort is often rewarded with the heightened personal insight they achieve in a private discussion with the instructor. The dialogue teaches students how to accept constructive criticism and provide specific feedback and data on their performance.

INSTRUCTOR EVALUATION OF THE STUDENT

One of the most important aspects of clinical care coordination is evaluation (Potter, Perry, Stockert, & Hall, 2013). This principle logically extends to evaluation of care rendered by nursing students. Once you are hired by the nursing program, your initial orientation to the clinical instructor role should include a detailed explanation of the procedure

Exhibit 9.1

Student Self-Evaluation of Clinical Performance

Grading Methodology

Grading for performance at the clinical site will follow the (*course name or number can appear here*) evaluation tool.

This self-evaluation is your opportunity to comment on your clinical performance. The grade range is a 1 to 5 Likert scale, which is defined as follows:

1. Does not meet clinical criteria
2. Is inconsistent in meeting clinical criteria
3. Meets clinical criteria
4. Exceeds clinical criteria
5. Far exceeds clinical criteria

Example Objective

"Attend each clinical session and submit required materials."

If your daily performance and submitted materials meet the expected standard, you may assign yourself a 3. If you exceed these minimum requirements, you may award yourself a 4 or 5, but you must provide *written* evidence for this elevated grade. Keep a log of any instances where you performed above minimum criteria. You cannot rate yourself higher than a 3 if you do not provide the written evidence for that grade. Submit this evidence with your self-evaluation. In the context of this example, here are some ways to exceed clinical criteria and achieve a grade above 3:

- Arrive on the unit early to read your patient's chart and to ask pertinent questions at the 7 a.m. preconference.
- Submit more than the minimum requirement of one journal per week. Incorporate classroom objectives and knowledge.
- Present a clinically related topic of interest to peers or a patient.
- Conduct independent research regarding your patient's care.

Note: Self-evaluation grades higher than 3 that are not supported with written evidence of accomplishment will be reduced to 3.

---

used to evaluate each student's clinical performance. Your own careful explanation of the clinical evaluation tool, including specific examples, should occur at the outset to clearly establish the expectations you will have of your students as they navigate through their clinical experiences. Emphasize to your students that performance evaluations will be an ongoing process throughout their nursing careers. If your school uses grades in its clinical evaluation, it is even more important to spend time preparing for this feature of your job, as seen in Chapter 12. Many students today expect "A" grades. They may be entering the field of nursing with an agenda. Some will tell you they want to be nurse anesthetists, nurse practitioners, and so on. The pressure that individual students may feel (which will be transferred to you if you are not careful) is, "I need 'A' grades to get the high GPA that is required to achieve my chosen nursing role." Students may be accustomed to receiving "A" grades and see no reason for you to alter that trend. In this context, it is advisable to have documentation describing what it takes to achieve an "A." See the grading guide in Exhibit 5.3, which represents an instructor's own supplement to the course syllabus for a specific clinical rotation and was created in response to student requests.

Many students are seeking feedback and suggestions in their ongoing pursuit of competency in clinical nursing. This evaluation time can be one of the most important sessions of their entire nursing curriculum. Many of today's experienced nurses can cite an instance when a clinical instructor gave them positive or negative feedback during a clinical evaluation and the impact of those observations on their nursing careers.

STUDENT EVALUATION OF THE INSTRUCTOR

Many schools allow your clinical students to evaluate you—the instructor—at the end of each clinical rotation. This third review exists outside of the formal clinical course evaluation itself. Participation is voluntary, anonymous, and there is no subsequent discussion between students and the instructor. Schools that provide this opportunity to their students do so to assess instructor performance from the "customer" perspective. The instructor's involvement here is simply to deliver the survey instrument. Completed evaluations of the instructor are submitted online or to a designated location by the respondents for tabulation by program administration. If your school utilizes this type of input, the results can have a big impact if your tenure or continued part-time employment is dependent on favorable student evaluations. Often a 4-point Likert scale is used in conjunction with the following observations:

- Organizes and plans the course effectively
- Makes the goals of the course clear

- Interacts effectively with the students
- Treats students in a respectful manner
- Encourages students to ask questions and participate
- Is enthusiastic about the subject
- Is clear about instructions for assignments
- Grades students' work fairly

Usually, there is a blank space provided for students to freely describe the best features of the instructor and course, as well as the features that could be improved. Be kind to yourself when reading these evaluations. Most of the time you will be pleased by what the students have to say, but heed this advice. Anyone who teaches nursing students long enough will receive a negative rating or comment at some point. It may not be possible to properly do the job that you are being entrusted with and always get glowing student evaluations. Accept that your honest appraisal of deficient student clinical performance may result in backlash when that same student assesses your work. This is an "occupational hazard" that all instructors face, so do not feel that you are alone. It can help to talk over any negative evaluation with a trusted colleague. If comments are unfair and you fear consequences from your superiors, make an appointment with the coordinator of the course and explain the possible motivation of the particular student or group that rated you poorly. Remember that self-compassion and self-care are essential to maintain satisfaction in the role of clinical instructor (more about that in Chapter 19).

Ideally, you should use the students' evaluation of your performance as a source of input that can make you a better instructor. Some of their suggestions can actually be very good!

Essential Facts

- Student self-evaluation is a valuable tool.
- Guidelines that instruct students how to document their performances are recommended, particularly as they relate to "above-satisfactory" achievement.
- Students' self-evaluations, when compared with the instructor's assessment, are important opportunities for dialogue and feedback.

References

Gaberson, K. B., & Oermann, M. H. (2010). *Clinical teaching strategies in nursing* (3rd ed.). New York, NY: Springer Publishing.

Potter, P., Perry, A., Stockert, P., & Hall, A. (2013). *Fundamentals of nursing* (8th ed.). St. Louis, MO: Elsevier.

10

The *Dos* and *Don'ts* of Student Documentation

A common mistake that clinical instructors make in their student clinical evaluations often involves insufficient documentation. "Anecdotal notes" are useful as the traditional format to document clinical performance. However, more official documentation by the clinical instructor becomes imperative when the student's performance leaves him or her in jeopardy of not passing the course. This chapter illustrates examples of anecdotal notes. It also offers concrete directions on the type of data needed to document the evaluation in a timely way. In addition, it discusses how to use anecdotal notes to decrease nursing instructors' professional liability.

In this chapter, you will learn:

- How to document "anecdotal notes"
- Key aspects of documentation pertinent to the clinical instructor
- The need for nursing instructors to understand their professional liability

DOCUMENTING STUDENT PERFORMANCE

The clinical instructor's assessment of student performance is an ongoing process. The student evaluation should reflect a compilation of observations in this process. Ensuring that the student evaluation presents a fair picture of performance requires avoiding common mistakes of judgment, so let's look at these "Don'ts" first.

The Don'ts

As a new instructor:

- *Don't* adopt a casual approach to documenting a student's clinical performance.
- *Don't* depend on "remembering" the specifics of each student's experiences when (a) administering medications; (b) assessing patients; (c) teaching patients; and (d) interacting with staff, their peers, or even with you!
- *Don't* think that because the student is hanging an intravenous medication or inserting a urinary catheter for the first time, mistakes should be disregarded because of a lack of preparation.
- *Don't* conclude that little harm or injury will ensue after a student encounter, such as patient assessment, even though the nurse stated that the patient was "upset" that day.
- *Don't* assume that the instructor has no financial or legal risk associated with student errors because students carry their own liability insurance.

The Dos

Be cautious. Too casual of an approach to documenting a student's clinical performance can lead to a final student evaluation that cannot be supported. The instructor may "feel" that a student adequately performed during a specific clinical rotation but did not exceed the minimum expectation of the clinical program. That student may, quite possibly, have an entirely different perspective. The student may believe that he or she performed in an exemplary manner and can cite specific examples in his or her self-evaluation. Unless the instructor has maintained an organized file of "anecdotal notes" to refute this perception, the instructor's assessment may face a student's challenge that can often involve extensive follow-up and work by the instructor.

This may include discussions between the instructor and the level or course coordinator or school chairperson, as well as other assigned faculty members. There are usually procedures in place regarding these types of student issues. Each nursing program has a different procedure for handling student clinical course issues.

If an instructor depends on "remembering" the specifics of each student's experience, the student evaluation can be murky and irrelevant. With a number of students to evaluate, even a person with a sharp memory may have difficulty recalling the specifics of each student's performance, including the adequacy and degree to which various nursing skills were implemented and evaluated.

In evaluating students, never disregard "lack of preparation." If students have been notified that they will be administering medications and performing certain procedures, it is incumbent upon the students to prepare by practicing in the nursing lab. Clinical instructors often have minimal time to teach and review an entire procedure for a student, particularly if a patient is to receive treatment in a timely manner. Nursing labs are available in all nursing programs today. Many labs have actually been revised and updated to incorporate high-fidelity simulation experiences (see Chapter 21 for more information). It is the students' responsibility to make arrangements to visit the lab and review necessary skills before their clinical experiences.

Make the nursing staff your ally. They have eyes and ears that can interpret and gather more information about your students' performance than you can obtain alone. If a staff nurse or nursing assistant mentions to you that a patient or a family seemed upset after the student performed a skill or entered the patient's room, *investigate*. This revelation often is a "red flag" that indicates a possible problem for the student, the school of nursing, and *you*. Go into the patient's room, introduce yourself to the patient and family, and ask how the student interaction was received by the patient. It is better to take care of any potential problem immediately rather than let it fester. Addressing it a week or two later may mean the difference between a prompt resolution and a legal situation.

Another helpful tip is to check with the nurse manager from time to time. This is being proactive as a teacher and evaluator. Go and inquire if there have been any concerns or issues. You may hear issues from patients or staff that fell through the cracks. However, checking in with the nurse manager will enhance your relationship with him or her and often earn you the goodwill of the nursing staff as well. When the nursing program submits its routine inquiries to clinical sites requesting placement for the upcoming semester, that unit will ask for you!

ANECDOTAL NOTES

As recommended in Chapter 2, be sure to understand your professional liability at the clinical site. Teachers and students are held to the same standards of care that a reasonably prudent person with the same level of education and experience would use in the same or similar circumstances (Lessner as cited in Oermann & Gaberson, 2013). The determination of professional liability can vary from state to state, and the appropriate state board of nursing can provide any specifics you may need. As a general rule, however, teachers are not liable for negligent acts performed by their students if they have done the following:

1. Selected appropriate learning activities based on skills necessary to complete the assignment.
2. Determined that the students have the necessary knowledge and skills to complete the assignment.
3. Provided necessary guidance.

To show that you, the clinical nursing instructor, have in fact complied with these requirements, it is helpful to devise a system for maintaining "anecdotal notes" relating to each student's performance. These notes are observations of a student's performance or behavior. See Exhibit 10.1 for an example.

Exhibit 10.1

Anecdotal Notes for Nursing 411 and NSL 412   Date: _____

Student	Performance aspect	Observation
Student #1		
Student #2		
Student #3		
Student #4		
Student #5		
Student #6		
Student #7		
Student #8		
Student #9		
Student #10		

There is a course title and date at the top. On the left side of the table, you can enter the name of each student. For each clinical day, document the performance aspect (e.g., a head-to-toe assessment or administration of a subcutaneous injection under your observation). These notes are for your eyes only and may prove invaluable in the unlikely event that your professional conduct relative to the three criteria is challenged! At the very least, your own notes during the day will help jog your memory when it is time for the clinical evaluation. They will be a great asset, especially after several weeks of a clinical practicum. You may also want to maintain a book with a separate page for each student—a copybook of sorts. Although the use of a notepad for this purpose may seem archaic, it can be a practical solution at clinical sites that prohibit the use of smartphones and lack the space for your tablet or laptop. After each clinical day, jot down a few notes about each student. An example of such a note might be:

> Mary administered Ancef IV and gave three oral medications to her patient. Her knowledge base of the oral medications was weak. I recommended to her that she write down pertinent facts about the meds before she contacts me saying she is prepared to give meds.

Writing such brief notes will help you identify whether a specific student followed your suggestion or repeated the same weak performance the next time that she was assigned to administer medications. If a particular student repeated the same substandard performance, it could be a "warning" sign. Discussion of warning signs for clinical instructors can be found in Chapter 11.

It is also helpful to keep a log of your comments regarding any written work submitted during the clinical practicum. For example, if weekly journals are due, devise a system to rate the journals and either write a number on each assignment or write your own note for each assignment in your own anecdotal notes. Today's students crave feedback, often and daily. By assigning a number (explain it in your own rating scale for evaluation purposes), you are giving them "feedback." Thoughts such as "needed much prompting on written journal in week 2 to include all categories of med classifications" will suffice to support your grading later in the semester. Keeping track of the number of each concept map or care plan is a chore that will be richly rewarded at evaluation times. Check in with the level or course coordinator regarding any written assignments. They may also have a grading rubric or grading form that can assist with the overall evaluation of the assignment.

Any system for keeping notes will do. Even an electronic record of this information is effective. The bottom line is that you need to write a note or two on each student each day of the clinical rotation, so take the time to document. The nursing profession teaches new students that if it is not documented, it did not happen. For a successful student evaluation, make sure that your anecdotal notes reveal what did happen.

Essential Facts

- Avoid the "mistakes" of a new clinical instructor regarding student evaluations.
- "Anecdotal notes" document a clinical instructor's daily attention to student performance.
- A written record of clinical performance is needed to support a student's weakness or failure.

Reference

Oermann, M. H., & Gaberson, K. B. (2013). *Evaluation and teaching in nursing education* (4th ed.). New York, NY: Springer Publishing.

11

Early Warning System

Many experienced clinical nursing instructors use a large amount of intuition when observing students. There are usually warning signs if a student is in jeopardy of not meeting the clinical objectives of the course. For example, a student may perform a nursing skill in a certain manner or communicate an aspect of the nursing process in such a way that the experienced instructor is alerted to a potential problem. Because nurses are charged with serious and potentially life-sustaining responsibilities, these sometimes subtle "warning signs" are important to heed and address. This chapter provides guidance about when it is prudent to contact your superiors and colleagues to assist you in this challenging task.

In this chapter, you will learn:

- How to identify the warning signs that a student may be in jeopardy of not passing or safely performing in the clinical setting
- Important tips to develop a "sixth sense," or intuition, to help determine which students are at risk for performing unsafe practices on patients
- When to contact your superiors to help determine which students are at risk—for your and your students' protection

EARLY WARNING SIGNS

As stated in Chapter 9, a mid-term evaluation is recommended for any clinical rotation that extends for at least 6 days. If the rotation is fewer than 6 days, a mid-term evaluation is difficult to adequately complete. However, an informal meeting between you and individual students may be prudent. The informal meeting might be as simple as a quick review of the evaluation form and your feedback regarding the student's performance to date. The meeting may also offer you the opportunity to discuss any early warning signs that you have observed in the student's performance.

CLINICAL OBJECTIVES

Assessing student performance at the clinical site can be a formidable task. The nursing instructor is not afforded the luxury of objective testing to measure student success. There is no fill-in-the-blank means of gauging the student's knowledge and safety on the floor and no multiple-choice test that can measure clinical effectiveness. Rather, the clinical teacher must base his or her judgment on direct observation within the context of written clinical objectives whose lack of precision can make them challenging to interpret. Examples of clinical objectives include the following:

- Demonstrates ability to meet the psychological needs of the critically ill patient.
- Interprets own verbal and nonverbal communications accurately.
- Demonstrates appropriate interactions with all patients.

Different nursing instructors can interpret these objectives in various ways. How does a novice clinical instructor decide what information to note for later use in evaluating student performance in terms of the program's objectives?

"RED FLAG" WARNINGS

There is another aspect to becoming an astute clinical instructor. This involves awareness of the more common "red flags" that students may wave during their clinical rotation—signals that warrant an instructor's observation, concern, consultation, and action plan.

Here are some examples of "warning signs":

- *Hedging:* Students who arrive unprepared sometimes will try to answer your questions by hesitantly bringing up many unrelated facts. An example of "hedging" is when the instructor asks the student to explain why a patient has intermittent compression devices on his legs after surgery. The student replies that it is for postoperative prevention of complications, but neither can the student specifically verbalize or describe the relevant complications that occur after surgery nor elaborate on nursing actions that prevent surgical complications. The student may offer other irrelevant details about the use of compression devices for orthopedic patients and the types of compression devices in the market. However, the student does not give a direct answer to your question. If the student does not know the specifics of why a nursing measure is taken, he or she cannot evaluate the effectiveness of the measure.
- *Late submission of assignments:* Students are given a timetable for completing their assignments, such as care plans, journals, and other assigned work. Students who submit their work late (on more than one occasion) may be having difficulty. It is possible that they have time constraints related to employment and may be working too many hours to complete their school work in a timely manner. They may not be conscious of the need for timeliness in a field where it is necessary to be on time with nursing care. Late assignment submissions often have a cause that you as the instructor should investigate. Do not just think that you are helping the student by "letting it go." The vital importance that the timely completion of tasks plays in the care of the patient must be instilled at the outset.
- *Late arrival at the clinical site:* Nursing care is an ongoing process in which the arriving nurse continues the flow of care rendered by his or her predecessor from the preceding shift. Lateness can greatly compromise this continuity. Students must clearly understand that being late for the clinical rotation is much more serious than being late for class. Unless the lateness is an unavoidable and isolated instance, such as a car accident, failure to appear at the designated hour is a very disconcerting sign. Do they really appreciate the tremendous responsibilities that accompany this profession? Are other parts of their lives interfering with their education? Whatever the cause, it is the clinical instructor's task to address the situation with the student,

review consequences for any continued lateness, and evaluate the student's ability to continue meeting the objectives of the course and the clinical instructor's expectations.

- *Absence on a clinical day:* Everyone gets sick and misses time from work or class occasionally. We are only human. Even so, students who miss more than a few hours of clinical time may deserve your concern. Missing hours repeatedly in multiple clinical rotations is a warning sign that students may not be able to cope with the demands of the field, and it may necessitate the involvement of the course coordinator and designated educational administrators. Nursing is not a solitary profession. The absence of one nurse on an assigned work day affects the entire team, and by extension, patient quality of care, which is why most hospitals and other health care organizations have absentee policies. It is imperative that each instructor should keep his or her supervisor apprised of all student absences. As mentioned in Chapter 5, do not say that there is "make-up" work that can be completed in the event of an absence (unless the program does in fact provide a make-up day at the end of the rotation for this purpose). Refer instead to an "alternate assignment" that can assist the student to meet the objectives missed that clinical day while acknowledging that there is no substitute for actual clinical experience (see Chapter 16).

- *Performing skills without supervision:* Chapter 5 provided information about the orientation day for the clinical instructor and new students. It was stated that upon arrival to a new hospital and unit, the rules and requirements of the host facility and school and the instructor's expectations should be provided in writing and reviewed. Noted in this review would be the instruction that "no nursing skill should be performed or medication given by the student without supervision." The instructor should clearly state who can provide such supervision. Will it always be you, or are there circumstances when the professional nurse in your host facility is permitted to supervise the student? Some instructors require that students sign a statement at orientation day that they understand these requirements. Incorporate this prudent practice in your own clinical oversight, because a student who performs a task or skill without the appropriate supervision can cause a serious and potentially deadly error. Should a breach of the supervision rule occur, it is paramount that you act immediately! Have a conference with the student that day, if possible right after the incident. You usually need to report this error to the unit floor manager and your contact person or coordinator at the school of nursing. Follow the school's policies in this regard (see Chapter 2) and also be aware of its "safe practice" criteria (see Chapter 17).

- *Chronic personal crises:* Every instructor knows that "life happens." Anyone can have a bad day or perform in a manner that is not optimal. At the same time, be aware of the student who continually offers excuses for less-than-stellar clinical performance. For example, all students may be advised by the instructor to visit their nursing lab before the start of the clinical practicum in order to review certain procedures, such as insulin injections or administering medications through a feeding tube. If you notice that a particular student clearly does not know which step to take first to perform this required skill, obviously the student's preparation is not adequate. The student may offer reasons for poor performance, ranging from physical illness to emotional heartbreak. At first, many instructors will extend the benefit of the doubt and walk the student through the procedure. This forgiving approach, however, should include advising the student that the lack of preparation indicates that more review time is warranted with the lab coordinator and should be accompanied by appropriate documentation in the anecdotal notes. However, if you observe the same lack of preparation in the same student a second time, you have received a "warning sign."

TAKING ACTION ON WARNING SIGNS

What should the clinical instructor do about these warning signs? If you are relatively new to the field of clinical instruction, discuss these observations with a more experienced colleague. Clinical instructors develop their own methodologies for working with students. Courtesy would indicate that you notify the lab instructor in advance as to what you expect from the lab time. You may then send the student to the nursing lab with a written instruction of what specifically occurred during the clinical time. You may request a written note or e-mail notification from the lab instructor confirming that the student did indeed complete the requested lab time. If enough warning signs accrue, the student may be in jeopardy of failing the clinical course. Familiarize yourself with the performance evaluation form and follow some of the suggestions in documenting unsafe practice in Chapters 10 and 17.

The Importance of Including Your Level or Course Coordinator

Considering the cost of tuition and the life changes that each student makes to become a nurse, it is essential that you give him or her adequate warning and remediation opportunities as early as possible if there is even a remote possibility that he or she may not be successful in your clinical rotation. Do not hesitate to document your concerns about the student, perhaps using the form in Exhibit 11.1.

Exhibit 11.1

Sample Counseling Form

College of XYZ
Health Science Division
Counseling Form
NUR11L
Student Conference

Student:
Subject:
Date:
Time:
Present:

Areas of Discussion:

Plan of Action:

Student Comments:

_____   _____
Student   **Date**

_____   _____
Faculty/Clinical/Lab Instructor **Date**

_____   _____
Course Coordinator   **Date**

Taking no action in the hopeful belief that "it is early, they will improve" is a roll of the dice that may have you in a difficult and time-consuming situation at the rotation's end. Specifically, if you have not delivered a formal clinical warning in a timely manner to allow the student full opportunity to improve and meet the clinical objectives, your ability to assign a failing grade at the end of the clinical rotation may be hampered by the of lack supporting documentation.

So, if in Week 1, one of your students is unprofessional in his or her interactions with a nurse, patient, or yourself, document and discuss the particulars with your student and notify your coordinator in writing. It is a more fair and just system that offers early remediation plans to students to give them the opportunity to meet the objectives of each clinical rotation. Remember that the nursing field is not a profession for everyone and that hard truth as it relates to a given individual will usually reveal itself for the first time in the clinical setting. Caring alone does not create a competent nurse. If you accumulate evidence that a student may not be suited for the nursing profession, discuss this with your coordinator and inquire whether a meeting to discuss the student's appropriateness for the field is warranted. Ironically, it is ultimately a true kindness to have this difficult discussion with your student, but be prepared; it may not be appreciated at the time.

IMPORTANCE OF INTUITION

As you become a more experienced clinical instructor, you will rely more on your intuition. A student will impress you with some of his or her interactions with patients, and you will realize that you need not observe that student as keenly as others. These days, clinical instructors have a clinical group assignment with six to 10 students. With as many as 10 students, you need to develop a sense for determining which students need close scrutiny for patient safety and which are more competent in their skills.

Trust your instincts. You developed these similar instincts as a staff or primary nurse when you "just had a feeling" that the patient was not doing well, and you spent additional time with that patient. It will be the same with student nurses. In time, your own instincts will alert you to the students who have a greater potential of possibly causing injury to the patients in their care.

Essential Facts

- Be alert for warning signs in students' performance.
- If you observe a warning sign, document it and notify your course coordinator immediately.
- Trust your instincts concerning "problem students."

12

Graded Clinical Versus Pass/Fail Evaluations

The time constraint inherent in clinical teaching has been acknowledged in this book. This is what makes the job of clinical instructors a bit more challenging than what is typically faced elsewhere in academia. However, because the profession of nursing is seen as a practice discipline at its core, students must be evaluated according to how they practice and, therefore, "perform." Clinical students can be graded with pass/fail, satisfactory/unsatisfactory, letter/number grade, or a combination of these systems.

In this chapter, you will learn:

- How each grading system works
- The advantages and disadvantages of each system

GRADING STUDENTS

In clinical teaching, the evaluation is the most difficult and emotionally charged responsibility (Scanlon, Care, & Gressler, 2001). Clinical instructors must deal with degrees of subjectivity in evaluating another person's performance, as well as with the fact that they do not have much time to spend with, let alone evaluate, students!

Challenges in Evaluating Students

Clinical instructors are consistently faced with several challenges in evaluating student performance. In some programs, an entire clinical rotation may last only 2 weeks. Moreover, the instructor is responsible for not just one student, but a group of students! For example, in a generic nursing program, the clinical instructor may be responsible for written evaluations and grades for as many as 10 students after a 7-week medical–surgical rotation.

Remember that often in nursing courses, there will be a separate classroom grade and a separate clinical grade for one course. Usually, the student must pass both segments of the course to progress to the next step in the nursing program. There are some students who are superior test takers and do well in classroom courses, but this does not always mean that they will also do well in the clinical component of the course. Clinical nursing courses are the essential component of nursing education that allow each student to transfer and apply learned knowledge into real situations.

Knowledge of Course Objectives

Instructors observe and score a student's performance based on a set of critical criteria linked to the course objectives. Therefore, it is imperative that clinical instructors familiarize themselves with the clinical course objectives; set time for mid-term and final clinical evaluation periods; and, most importantly, be familiar with the grading system.

Unanticipated Events

In addition, anticipated and unanticipated events can affect the valuable time instructors have with students. For most clinical rotations, the first day is usually the assigned hospital orientation day. Other days may be lost to university or nursing program events that students are required to attend or legal holidays on which classes are canceled. Unanticipated events, such as extreme weather conditions or school disasters, may result in school closure. All of these events affect the number of days instructors have for observing and evaluating student performance.

TYPES OF GRADING SYSTEMS

The grading system for clinical courses is primarily based on the student's achievement of certain course objectives. Clinical courses are usually offered on a pass/fail grading system or letter/number grading system. See Exhibit 12.1 for a commonly used grading system that could be found in any student handbook.

Pass/fail grades and satisfactory/unsatisfactory grades are synonymous and do not provide comparative gradations among passing students. A letter grade offers a finer evaluation of a student's performance. Grading is usually specific to the nursing program. Exhibit 12.2 is another example of a grading system that would be found in a clinical course. In clinical teaching, the pass/fail grading basis predominates. A national study referenced in *Nursing Education Perspectives* found that 83% of surveyed faculty utilize the pass/fail grading method (Oermann, Yarbrough, Saewert, Ard, & Charasika, 2009).

Exhibit 12.1

Grading System

The grading system used for nursing courses is based on the student's achievement of the course objectives. The grading scale is as follows:

Letter grade	Percentage grade	Quality points
A	93–100	4.0
B	84–92	3.0
C	75–83	2.0
F	Below 75	0.0

Exhibit 12.2

Nursing 3116 Advanced Adaptation Course

Nursing 3116 Clinical Course

Clinical Grading System: The grading system used for nursing clinical courses is based on the student's achievement of the course objectives. The grading scale is as follows:

Pass or Fail

The clinical component is graded as pass or fail. This means that you will not receive a letter grade for the course; rather, you will receive a grade of "P" for satisfactory work and "F" for unsatisfactory work. Pass grades are included in total credits earned but pass/fail grades are not included in the grade point average.

Satisfactory or Unsatisfactory (Pass/Fail)

The clinical rotation can be graded as satisfactory or unsatisfactory. A final grade of satisfactory is required in the clinical component of a nursing course. If the student is not demonstrating a pattern of satisfactory clinical performance, the clinical instructor will meet with the student to formulate a plan for improvement. Students must achieve all clinical course objectives/competencies by the end of the course to receive a satisfactory grade. An unsatisfactory clinical grade in any objective at the end of the course usually results in course failure regardless of grades received on classroom assignments, tests, and examinations. The final course grade will be recorded as an F.

CLINICAL EVALUATION FORMS

Clinical evaluation forms reflect the specific behavioral objectives of that course. To assist students in meeting these objectives, specific clinical criteria are established and written out clearly on the evaluation form. These clinical criteria are presented to the students and discussed with them on the first clinical day. The student's performance and the instructor's observations are the key elements in the evaluation process.

Evaluations of clinical criteria are clearly highlighted in the clinical evaluation tool and may be given orally to the student by the instructor during the evaluation time.

CLINICAL OBJECTIVE EXAMPLE

An example of a clinical objective is: *The student applies knowledge of medical–surgical nursing when providing patient care.*

An instructor using the pass/fail grading system would report a P (pass) or an F (fail) for this objective based on that student's performance in the setting. In a program using the letter/number grading system, the instructor would score the student based on the rating scale. The scale is usually a Likert-type scale ranging from 1 to 5. See the example in Chapter 9. The scale scores for each objective would then be tallied to give a final clinical score.

Essential Facts

- Each program defines its own clinical evaluation system.
- Clinical objectives are highlighted in the clinical evaluation tool.
- A 1-to-5 rating scale is commonly used in a letter/number clinical grading system.

References

Oermann, M. H., Yarbrough, S. S., Saewert, K. J., Ard, N., & Charasika, M. E. (2009). Clinical evaluation and grading practices in schools of nursing: National survey findings part II. *Nursing Education Perspectives*, *30*(6), 352–357.

Scanlon, J. M., Care, W. D., & Gressler, S. (2001). Dealing with the unsafe student in clinical practice. *Nurse Educator*, *26*(1), 23–27.

V

Managing the Clinical Day

13

Preconferences

Preconferences are preclinical meetings held at the start of a clinical day. These conferences are led by a clinical instructor and can provide teaching and learning opportunities. These allow the clinical instructor the opportunity to assess the student's preparation and assignment for the clinical day and to observe key aspects of the student's communication skills that are necessary to nursing practice. Communication competence is an essential nursing skill because of the daily interactions nurses have with patients and other health care providers. Proper preparation for the clinical day is also essential and is an evaluation objective for all levels of nursing students.

In this chapter, you will learn:

- The value and proper use of preconference time
- The role of the preconference in relation to the objectives of the nursing process. One scenario of a type of preconference will be highlighted

WHAT IS A PRECONFERENCE?

During the clinical rotations, the instructor will schedule conferences. These conferences are usually held before the start of a clinical day and are called preconferences. If scheduled at the end of the day, they are called postconferences. For the clinical faculty, these conferences are a teaching–learning strategy because they are expected to follow up on elements from the classroom lectures. They also use these conferences to plan learning opportunities for their students—ones that will assist the student with the primary goal of "application of theory into practice."

STUDENT GUIDANCE

Each clinical instructor should remember that no one else is giving these students direction about the specific clinical rotation. Instructors are responsible for providing all guidance and addressing all questions regarding all aspects of the clinical experience. Their job responsibilities include setting the rules and structuring the clinical day according to the objectives of the course and program. Although students should learn the majority of the rules and instructors' expectations on orientation day, conferences with students during the rotation also provide opportunities to share expectations and reinforce clinical guidelines.

Daily Expectations

Students will become frustrated if they do not know what is expected of them each clinical day. Students should not be surprised about the rules and guidelines or arrive at a hospital unit without adequate preparation from the instructor. What kind of "preparation" is the clinical instructor responsible for? Instructors must clarify behaviors that are expected of their students. It is recommended that instructors do this by giving clear examples of satisfactory and unsatisfactory performance using the clinical evaluation tool as their guide. This also requires clarifying the clinical objectives set forth by the nursing program, which are usually broad and unspecific in relation to the actual elements of patient care. Each student needs to know the specific elements of patient care for which he or she will be responsible and the general timeline of each clinical day. This can best be done during a preconference.

Patient Care Assignments

The students usually receive their patient care assignments at this time. Many instructors are allowing students more latitude in choosing their patients for the day. If you give clear directions about which type of patient is best for the student to meet the objectives, the student can play the major role in choosing his or her patients with guidance from you and the unit's nursing staff. Remember your job is to foster independence and some sense of self-efficacy for each student. Use every opportunity to do so. If he or she receives the patient assignment before the preconference, the clinical instructor can review each student's plan of care during the preconference. In essence, the purposes of a preconference are to give faculty an opportunity to prepare the students for the clinical day, to review any work from the students, and to set the structure of the clinical day to avoid frustration for all parties. An example of a preconference scenario is provided in Exhibit 13.1.

In some programs, clinical instructors are expected to visit the site in advance of the clinical day to review and select patients for students, so that students can receive patient care assignments before the clinical day. If this is the expectation of your nursing program, then the preconference format may be structured differently than the preceding scenario. The preconference time can then be used to evaluate students' understanding of patients' medical diagnosis, medical history, nursing care plan, and priority nursing goals to make sure the students are adequately prepared. The preconference time can also be used as a teaching opportunity. The nursing instructor may highlight a certain class of medications, such as salicylates, and have the students discuss its interactions and side effects. In addition, student communication skills may also be observed and evaluated. The instructor can

Exhibit 13.1

Preconference Scenario

At orientation day, Jason, the clinical instructor, informed students that at the beginning of each clinical day, at 6:30 a.m. sharp, he would hold a preconference with the group in the cafeteria meeting room. The purpose was to give them the three learning goals for the clinical day, as well as to give each of them their patient care assignment. At one particular preconference, Jason shared the following goals for students to fulfill on that clinical day: (a) to complete an assessment of their patients, (b) to document that assessment, and (c) to understand the medication list for each patient. Students were given these goals orally and on a written handout from the instructor. In addition, one student, Nancy, received a patient in room 550, a 10-year-old patient with cystic fibrosis. The clinical instructor then directed Nancy and all the students to review the medical diagnosis and its medical and nursing management during the rest of the preconference time. Students were told to bring their textbooks or program-provided computer tablets to assist them with their preconference work.

inform students that preconference time will begin with each student stating his or her patient's initials, the diagnosis, medical and nursing management, and nursing goals.

When students receive patient care assignments in advance of the clinical day, the expectations are a bit different. There are higher expectations at the preconference and postconference because the students have more resources and time to prepare for the clinical day. Thus, the manner in which patient care assignments are distributed plays a role in the structure of the preconference session. However, throughout the clinical rotation, clinical faculty use these preconference sessions as evaluation opportunities to assess students' preparation for clinical days and to review their knowledge of the nursing process.

Essential Facts

- The structure of the clinical nursing preconference is determined by the timing of the patient assignments.
- For the clinical instructor, the preconference is a time for teaching and learning opportunities.
- The preconference can also be used to evaluate each student's preparation and assessment of his or her patient assignment.

14

Postconferences

Postconferences are held at the conclusion of a clinical day. Students are usually expected to present their patients at the postconference. This time allows the instructor to address any events that may have occurred during the clinical day.

In this chapter, you will learn:

- The purpose of postconferences
- An explanation of their importance to the overall learning objectives of the clinical course and the analysis of patient care

WHAT IS A POSTCONFERENCE?

Preconferences and postconferences are similar. They are both meeting times at which clinical issues are discussed and questions about clinical objectives are answered by the instructor. In addition, postconference time is also seen by many as the best time for students to "debrief" about the events during their day. Debriefing is defined as an information-sharing event that consists of a conversation between peers (Hanna & Romana, 2007). To differentiate between the two conference times, most clinical faculty will lead the preconference but follow the students' lead at the postconference. The reason is primarily associated with the timing of the conference. The conclusion of a long clinical day provides a better opportunity for the instructor to ascertain students' understanding of their patients' care and to question students about their findings from the chart and their own patient assessment.

TEACHING OPPORTUNITIES

Clinical faculty can use postconferences as opportunities for teaching and student learning. As such, the clinical instructor can, for example, review lab values with the clinical group at one postconference session. Or the postconference can be used to link class theory with actual practice elements. For example, if the class topic is respiratory obstructive disorders, during postconference, the instructor can elaborate on the lab values associated with this class of disorders. Or the postconference can focus on respiratory acidosis and the role played by arterial blood gases. In general, most postconference times are focused learning events about the nursing process, fundamental concepts, or any patient education principles. For example, the clinical instructor may have students review the Internet resources provided as resources for patients and their families. You may also find some clinical instructors giving a "mini-test" about certain nursing care principles they want enforced. Most clinical faculty will plan many learning activities for their students. One such activity is student presentations.

Student Presentations

Students can be assigned a 10-minute presentation on a nursing topic appropriate to the objectives of the clinical rotation. These student presentations can also be viewed as a communication assignment. Another assigned learning activity can relate to literature review, evidence-based practice, and writing. Depending on the level of students, the clinical instructor can collect literature reviews on research studies related to the course objectives or have students conduct an actual review on current evidence-based practice related to a particular topic. Students can then verbalize some aspects of this search and present the findings during postconference.

Students can also be encouraged to review the NCSBN-RN® exam blueprint during postconference time. At that time, they can review how their topic fits into the National Council of State Boards of Nursing (NCSBN) main content categories and subcategories. It is always a good idea to expose student nurses to the NCSBN website (www.ncsbn.org) and the blueprint in order to get them thinking of the license exam that they will have to complete for licensure. The NCSBN-RN® license blueprint can be found at this website (www.ncsbn.org/RN_Test_Plan_2016_Final.pdf).

Clinical instructors can also use this blueprint for a writing exercise. They can have students write two or three exam questions on a particular topic. For example, if the postconference discussion was about an issue with informed consent, then students can be directed to develop exam questions on informed consent. Like a preconference, postconferences can take up to 1 hour. Because of these time limitations, clinical instructors must be organized and designate any postconference assignment from the start. It is also wise to provide students with an assigned due date for each learning assignment.

Understand Conference Limitations

Do not overwhelm the conference time by including too many teaching–learning opportunities. Always be true to your students and be in touch with their psychosocial well-being. At the end of a clinical day during which they have been continuously evaluated, they are mentally and physically exhausted. *Know their limits.* This important tip will keep you from being frustrated as you set your own expectations for the postconference.

SHARING STUDENT EXPERIENCES

One word of caution about these conferences. Although clinical instructors often use preconferences and postconferences as an evaluation opportunity, not all conferences should be seen as evaluation time. The effective clinical instructor will also hold conferences that are devoid of the evaluation "hat." Such conferences allow students to share experiences and interact with the group without the stress of performance evaluation or the knowledge that a comment or action will be documented in their clinical evaluation. Inform your students when they will be specifically evaluated. Allow for free sharing of experiences. Once you do that, your conferences will run smoothly and will meet your expectations. If you choose, you can use the first 10 minutes of a postconference to ascertain any moments of anxiety or to gauge reactions to certain skills the students performed. You may want to start with an open-ended question, such as "For those who gave medications today, what are your thoughts and feelings about the experience?"

Because many teaching and learning opportunities exist, the clinical instructor should be cautioned not to try too many at once. Remember that postconferences can be a productive time for teaching and learning, a time when students have an opportunity to address concerns or voice issues regarding their patient care or their performance. Students may also question something that happened during the course of a day. Addressing concerns and questioning an event that may have occurred are examples of debriefing.

Sample Scenario

Exhibit 14.1 provides an example of an appropriate event to discuss at a postconference. As this scenario illustrates, the student's assessment findings and the actions by the primary nurse can be a key discussion point for the postconference. In this scenario, the student verbalized key aspects of the patient's condition with the clinical group and shared the events that unfolded during care of the patient. Students in this clinical group had many questions regarding the patient's diet and whether this could have been a factor related to the hypoglycemia.

Lessons Learned From the Scenario

This example offers many good observation points about this particular student. The student was able to effectively verbalize the event and share the experience with the group. Debriefing occurred as classmates questioned each other. The student in the scenario was comfortable with these questions because there was a solid exchange of

Exhibit 14.1

Postconference Discussion Point

An undergraduate student in a progressive care unit was caring for a female patient recovering from open heart surgery and the complications of pneumonia. The patient could not speak because of a tracheostomy tube and was breathing room air. This was the second day the student was assigned to this patient. Knowing the patient from the previous day, the student noticed that the patient seemed more lethargic and became diaphoretic as she was completing the noon vital signs. The clinical instructor observed the student as she reported her findings to the assigned primary nurse. The blood glucose was quickly checked and revealed that the patient was acutely hypoglycemic. The primary nurse then alerted the physician.

thoughts and ideas in the group. More importantly, the clinical instructor observed the student's keen assessment of the patient as well as the student's actions of critical thinking (rechecking vital signs) and then the appropriate reaction (verbalizing the assessment concerns to the primary nurse). The student met many clinical objectives on this clinical day, from professional communication, to prioritizing data, to applying aspects of the nursing process in a safe and competent manner appropriate for the setting.

Clinical instructors will find that time to actually stop and teach is limited during the course of a clinical day. The day progresses so quickly that many key events come and go without time to "pause" to share a key aspect of care or highlight a particular intervention. The time to do this is at postconference. When there is something to be emphasized, an item to be taught, or an event to debrief, postconferences provide the time to share and discuss experiences.

Essential Facts

- Postconference time should not be directed by the instructor. Rather, it is a time to debrief about the aspects of the day.
- Have postconferences without wearing the evaluation "hat."
- Postconferences can be used as teaching and learning opportunities.

Reference

Hanna, D. R., & Romana, M. (2007). Debriefing after a crisis. *Nursing Management, 28*(8), 38–42, 44–45, 47.

15

Unplanned Events and Absences

As any nurse or professional will tell you, the world of health care is filled with unexpected or unanticipated moments. In fact, aside from the nursing process itself, there is nothing "routine" in health and illness. Relay this to your students, who may be expecting to find the same patient in the same condition every day. Each clinical course runs for a specific number of clinical hours and days, so that competencies are maintained. Students are required to arrive on time and be present each and every clinical day. Anticipating unplanned events, such as sleeping through an alarm, low census on the unit, acute changes in a patient's condition, resident outings, or patient discharges, is key to providing the best learning experience for the student.

In this chapter, you will learn:

- How to anticipate or plan in advance for changes in a student's clinical assignment
- How to develop a "toolbox" of potential alternate assignments that will save time when unplanned events occur
- The impact of absences and lateness on meeting clinical objectives

PLANNING ASSIGNMENTS

It is sometimes impossible to predict the census or patient composition of the clinical unit to which your students have been assigned during their rotation. It may also be difficult to predict which patients will be available for your students to interact with at a retirement facility, daycare setting, or school. How can you, as the clinical instructor, plan an assignment for your charges and also ensure that your students are meeting their learning objectives for the clinical course?

First, you have to create a student nurse clinical assignment. Think of all of the potential clinical placements in which today's student nurses may find themselves. Students are at nursery schools, senior centers, maternity units, and community settings, to name a few. Thus, the development of a solid clinical assignment encompasses the patients in the clinical setting as well as awareness of the knowledge level and familiarity with nursing practice of the current groups of students in your practicum. This can be the most challenging task faced by all clinical instructors, especially during the first few weeks of the clinical rotation when you are just starting to distinguish each student and to begin assessing "high" versus the "not-so-high" fliers. Listed next are some standard guidelines that clinical instructors can use in all settings.

GUIDELINES FOR CLINICAL ASSIGNMENTS

- *Be familiar with the student evaluation tool,* which will list the clinical objectives.
- *Use this tool as your "roadmap"* for developing assignments.
- *Develop a relationship with the nursing staff* at your facility so its members can assist you.
- *Accept the nursing staff's hints and suggestions.* Their input is invaluable. For example, a staff nurse may tell you, "That patient is not good for a student." *Heed their advice.* They know. They will know that the patient has an anxious family who would be hesitant to allow a student nurse to care for their relative. They will also know the patient who may be too threatening for a novice student.
- *Arrive a few hours before your students.* Arriving earlier will help you organize the clinical student assignment and provide time to talk to the staff and review the charts.

- *Review the end-of-shift or nursing report.* Find out if certain patients would appreciate a student, and learn those patients' schedules for that day. Will they be off of the unit most of the day for tests? Are they in too much pain to talk with the students on a day when a primary objective is oral communication?
- *Avoid writing down all the patient data.* It is not your role to communicate this detailed level of information to students. Part of the learning experience—and an essential component of your evaluation of each student—is students' understanding of what information is essential and where to locate that information. See Appendix C, a sample of brief data that can be shared with students electronically via an e-mail message or can be posted in an online classroom environment (commonly found in most nursing programs). Refer to the details found in Chapter 6 on patient privacy and maintaining confidentiality. Ensure that patient confidentiality is maintained when communicating via e-mail. This means that no patient names are allowed.
- *Be cognizant of each student's strengths and weaknesses.* For example, a student who has some initial self-confidence issues may not be the one to take on the cantankerous older adult patient who will "order" the student around all day. Students who are able to handle more difficult patients may appropriately receive a higher grade or be given a more positive evaluation than other students.
- *Be flexible.* The most detailed and well-prepared assignment may fall apart when patients are not available on the scheduled day or are unable to accept a student for some reason. A sense of humor will serve you well on these days.

When a clinical instructor is developing the assignments for that clinical day, an unplanned event such as student lateness on arrival or a student absence can affect the organization of the day. For example, if a specific student is scheduled to perform dressing changes on the unit that day but that student is absent, then the instructor must re-manage the assignment in order to optimize the experiences for the entire clinical group. There are also instances where a student arrives late due to road conditions or a personal issue. The discussion about having a backup plan will always save the instructor with untimely occurrences that can affect well-laid plans.

UNPLANNED EVENTS

Although most learning opportunities are planned in a clinical rotation, in acute care settings where illness, death, and various human experiences are the reality, you can be sure that "unplanned" events will likely occur. Try to have a "backup" plan when creating a student assignment. This can be accomplished by carrying with you relevant clinical case studies to use if circumstances result in a student's inability to complete objectives on a given day. For example, the student may have planned to perform a psychosocial assessment on the assigned client, but that patient has unexpectedly left for the day. The staff states that no other patient is available. This is an opportune time to give the student the case studies you are carrying, with the objective of reviewing and then presenting them to his or her peers at a postconference.

Another example of an unplanned event could be the student who arrives late because of a personal issue or road conditions. You can always assign two students to care for one patient in this instance. Thus, the one student has already started patient care and the other, upon arrival, can finish up using the nursing process. Working together teaches students that helping one another is essential to the practice of nursing. Often, students learn best from a peer because of the perceived nonthreatening manner of classmates, which may be of benefit to all.

BASIC COMPETENCIES IN THE CLINICAL SETTING

Students are assigned functions and responsibilities that are necessary to pass each clinical rotation. These rotations take place in various work environments, such as public health and community agencies, homes, schools, clinics, hospitals, and nursing homes. General responsibilities and assigned functions encompass those required for nursing practice and may include assessing patients, planning and delivering care, performing acute care interventions, providing direct care safely, teaching patients and their family members, and teaching community residents about health and illness. Students must also be competent in reviewing a patient's medical condition, summarizing the patient's chart, assessing health and illness, carrying out the physician's orders, and communicating with all parties. These are basic competencies for students in clinical settings.

To evaluate individual student performances, a certain number of days and a set number of hours are for the clinical instructor's review.

Even then, clinical instructors often find that the clinical rotation time is too short. Therefore, *instructors frown on student absences or tardiness* because it further minimizes the time available for student evaluation. Instructors are responsible for enforcing all policies pertaining to this conduct.

EFFECT OF TARDINESS ON CLINICAL OBJECTIVES

As with absences, the *clinical instructor and course coordinator should monitor student tardiness from the first day* of the clinical experience. Students can be tardy for numerous reasons, such as car problems and road conditions. However, the student should not offer these excuses to explain a pattern of tardiness. If a student arrives late every Tuesday morning, then the student has a responsibility problem and should be evaluated accordingly.

Each time a student is tardy, the instructor should be informed as early as possible. As soon as the student arrives, he or she must immediately seek out the clinical instructor for a briefing on what was missed. The clinical instructor can usually assign a late-arriving student to work with another student or to shadow a staff member (with the staff member's permission). Such adjustments depend upon the location of the clinical experience, because student responsibilities and duties vary by setting. If a student has a pattern of lateness, that student will probably not meet some of the clinical objectives.

EFFECT OF ABSENCES ON CLINICAL OBJECTIVES

The nursing program has a set policy regarding absences that is strictly enforced. Clinical instructors are told to inform the course coordinator of any student absence and to seek the assistance of the course coordinator regarding habitual policy violators. Most nursing programs have set mechanisms and procedures that clearly identify what students have to do in the event of a clinical absence. Most absences warrant evidence, such as documentation of illness from a health care provider.

At times, students become so fearful of being absent that they will come to the clinical rotation when they are ill because they are fearful of upsetting their clinical instructor, or because they are anxious and confused about the policy and procedures. But they may be very sick. You will look at them and then send them home. And in some instances, your students may become sick during the clinical day. The authors have had multiple students who have either fainted or became physically ill during the course of the day. If this occurs on site, the student should be sent to the emergency department and the clinical instructor should follow up with him or her and contact any family as appropriate. Usually the procedure is to also inform the course coordinator; he or she will thereby contact the nursing program and school administrators who need to be informed. Sound judgment and student safety are paramount in these situations.

All this discussion about the policy and the specific procedure should be discussed with students prior to arrival or on the first day of the clinical practicum. The student is primarily responsible for *informing the instructor* of an illness the night before or on the day of the clinical experience. Because of these possible situations, it is routine for clinical faculty to share their cell phone number with clinical students. However, they need to stipulate that this cell phone is only for professional use for the duration of the course.

For a prolonged and unexpected student absence, the routine procedure is for the assigned faculty to discuss the situation and designate a plan of action for that student. Most schools handle these situations on a case-by-case basis. Each case requires individual attention by the designated faculty. Clinical instructors are never alone in making these decisions.

Essential Facts

- Preparation for student assignments will often prove beneficial.
- Unplanned events will occur despite your best plans.
- Flexibility and a positive relationship with the staff at your facility will assist you in adapting a student assignment.
- Nursing programs have strict policies regarding absences and tardiness.

16

Alternative Assignments

All levels of students (from first to final year) will benefit from assignments "outside" of the specified clinical rotation. Supplemental experience in a department other than the assigned one enhances the educational value of the clinical site. This alternative assignment can occur in the community or pediatric, maternity, psychiatric, or medical–surgical rotations of a student's clinical experience. As noted in Chapter 15, it is helpful to have a plan for the "unplanned events" that inevitably occur on many clinical days. This chapter presents samples of alternative assignments based on the particular clinical rotations. They are accompanied by tips on methods for coordinating and cultivating these alternative assignments to benefit all parties, but especially the students.

In this chapter, you will learn:

- The value of providing alternative assignments for your students
- Sample alternative assignments for many different clinical rotations that instructors can use immediately in their current work
- Alternative assignments can be used for absences or for students who are out for prolonged periods

ALTERNATIVE ASSIGNMENTS RELATED TO ABSENCES

For minor illnesses, alternative assignments are provided to students on a course-by-course basis. However, there are nursing programs that allow students to make up the clinical experience on other days, either with the regular clinical instructor or another instructor. Students are required to pay "out of pocket" for this make-up time (based on a set fee structure). Other programs routinely prefer to provide alternative assignments for students. Examples of such work can be a critique of a research article, a presentation of a literature review, or the completion of several case studies from a workbook. This work should be collected within a week of the absence. It is wise to check with the program's course coordinator for other examples of acceptable make-up work.

At this time, most schools have turned to simulations as alternative assignments if they have a designated simulation lab area designed for simulation learning. At one school, the hospital site was overbooked and student access was denied 1 week before the start of the pediatric clinical rotation. With a simulation coordinator and simulation personnel, the course coordinator was able to move part of the clinical experiences to simulation labs with simulation experiences and the use of pediatric cases. Other worthwhile assignments may be extracted from this environment. Chapter 21 provides further discussion on the role of simulation in clinical education.

Clinical instructors should define and identify examples of alternative clinical work in their syllabi, thereby informing students of how these assignments can relate to meeting the required clinical objectives. If you need to devise and create alternative work, it is wise to have students complete assignments related to the clinical practicum or related to the nursing theory (didactic) course in which they are currently enrolled. Exhibits 16.1 and 16.2 offer examples of alternative assignments that can be applied to student groups.

MEETING PROGRAM OBJECTIVES

In all types of nursing programs—associate, diploma, or baccalaureate—the "guiding light" of your clinical rotations are the clinical objectives specified on the evaluation tool. Some schools use generic objectives that can be applied to multiple locations, such as maternity, pediatric, or psychiatric nursing settings. Other schools may have different objectives for each specific rotation. No matter the

Exhibit 16.1

Examples of Written Assignments for Clinical Absence

1. The instructor will assign a literature review on a medical–surgical nursing topic. The paper will be graded on the content and the format required for a literature review.

    The literature review will include a title page and a reference page (current). It will be a minimum of six pages, with the format and margins as required by the latest edition of the *Publication Manual of the American Psychological Association* guidelines.

    Due date: 10 days from absence.
2. The instructor will assign three case studies to be completed by the following Thursday.

Exhibit 16.2

Oral Assignments for Clinical Absence

Guidelines for an ethical–legal presentation:

1. Select an ethical or legal topic from the pediatric or medical–surgical nursing specialties as the basis for a discussion or debate.
2. Review the literature and provide a 5-minute presentation (including a written outline to be shared with the group) using one of the following techniques:
   - Focus on a recent debate issue.
   - Highlight a recent news item on the issue.
   - Present the research problem and identify a question.
   - Present a case study from your experience.
   - Summarize the literature.
3. Lead a 5-minute discussion on this topic.
4. Bonus points: any creativity brought to the presentation.

evaluation tool, instructors must follow these objectives and plan opportunities for all students to meet each program objective. This is often challenging. Remember that you may have up to 10 students in your rotation, and each must be given an equal opportunity to meet the required objectives. For this reason, it is prudent to develop "alternative assignments for specialties." These are not like the alternative assignments that may be used for a student absence or due to loss of a clinical site, but rather related to the complexities of your clinical rotation and the high student ratio that you may have.

ALTERNATIVE ASSIGNMENTS AT AN ALTERNATE SITE

These alternative assignments serve many purposes. They offer a chance to carry the stated purpose and knowledge of this rotation to a different location, where the student can often interact with different staff personnel. Another purpose of these alternative assignments is to create a more manageable number of students for you to evaluate and supervise on any given day. For example, an instructor has 10 students on an acute pediatric hospital unit to supervise. Several of these students need to administer medications, and all need to complete comprehensive patient care. This is a formidable task for any instructor. If two or three alternative assignments were created that met some of the clinical objectives of this pediatric rotation, then the instructor would have only seven nursing students on the acute care floor instead of 10.

Appropriate Assignments

An important caveat to these alternative assignments: They need to facilitate the students' attempts to meet their clinical objectives and the course coordinator needs to agree with your assessment of this alternative as safe and beneficial. An example of how these assignments can be abused or deemed inappropriate is shown in Exhibit 16.3.

Table 16.1 illustrates some possible alternative assignments for students in different rotations. Each instructor needs to modify these suggestions to his or her school's specifications and requirements.

Clinical Rotation Assignments

These are only a few of the creative and valuable alternative assignments that you can have in your repertoire. You must also give students clear instructions with each alternative assignment. For example, the student who spends the day with the pediatric nurse practitioner during his or her pediatric rotation must have a written format with objectives and requirements for that day.

Importance of Feedback

A written assignment describing how the aforementioned objectives were or were not fulfilled during that student's day may be required. It is also advisable to get feedback from the nurse practitioner about the student's performance. Exhibit 16.4 provides an example of instructions for an alternative assignment.

Exhibit 16.3

Inappropriate Alternative Assignment

Megan, a new nursing clinical instructor, supervised nine students for a 4-day rotation through an acute psychiatric unit. At an orientation session, the course coordinator communicated the clinical objectives to this instructor. The school has used this site for many years, and the school and unit nurses had a good working relationship.

Megan decided unilaterally that nine students were too many to supervise at one site. Without asking the level or course coordinator, she asked the facility's emergency department (ED) if she could send two students to the ED on each of the 3 clinical days and three students on a fourth day. All would therefore have the same opportunity.

The students reported this practice to the coordinator. The students were concerned about missing the needed opportunity to care for patients and meet their assigned objectives on an acute psychiatric unit. Because this was only a 4-day rotation, their concern was well founded. They all enjoyed the ED experience but knew that they were not meeting their primary objectives.

The level or course coordinator called the new instructor; they met privately to review the course and clinical objectives. The course coordinator also reminded the clinical instructor to keep all students on the acute psychiatric unit as prescribed by the nursing curriculum. Megan was asked why she had assigned these students to an alternative placement such as the ED during their brief psychiatric rotation. She responded that she thought students would have an opportunity to observe patients who came to the ED when in acute psychiatric crisis. Although there was a possibility that this could occur, it was unlikely. Moreover, Megan is now aware that she is required to check with the level or course coordinator before any alternative assignment was created.

Table 16.1

Samples of Possible Alternative Assignments

Clinical Rotation	Alternative Assignment
Acute hospital pediatric floor	Day with a pediatric nurse practitioner
Maternity rotation in hospital	Visit to a free-standing birth center
Acute psychiatric rotation	Visit to an outpatient community mental health center
Medical–surgical floor	Day in the critical care unit
Community health	Day at a migrant farm location

Exhibit 16.4

Assignments for Clinical Rotations

During your experience with the pediatric nurse practitioner, you will be concentrating on Objectives 1, 2, and 3 of your evaluation tool, which read:

1. Observe the role of each nurse in his or her relationship with ill children and in performing nursing responsibilities.
2. Familiarize yourself with the Nurse Practice Act and observe the nurse's extended role as a practitioner.
3. Assess the nursing process used with each pediatric patient during your experience.

Some examples of negative feedback would be:
"The student just sat in the corner of the office and read through journals."
"I attempted to engage the student and often pointed out different assessment findings, but the student just looked, said little, and returned to a corner seat."

This feedback is invaluable. These data could alert you to one of the early warning signals mentioned in Chapter 11. What is interfering with a student's ability to learn? Is it lack of motivation? Lack of sleep? Something is amiss, and it is now your opportunity to address the problem and try to correct it.

It is important that students do not view an alternative assignment as a "day off." Convey this information by carefully orienting students to the goals and written assignment for the day. Let the student know that you will talk to the nurses at the alternative assignment setting and receive feedback.

Prepare the Clinical Setting

As the clinical instructor, it is important to "scope" out the alternative assignment site and experience it for yourself before assigning a student. Verify that the nursing staff is willing to teach and have a student "shadow" them for the day. Be clear with the staff and management about the specifics of the student's assignment. For example, if the student is spending the day with the pediatric nurse practitioner, make sure that the student does not assess or document or perform any procedure while at the site. The student would probably not be covered for any liability if in a different locale or part of the clinical rotation. Stress that this is an observation experience only and be very clear with your students about the parameters of their responsibilities on that day.

Individualizing Student Assignments

Although there are general rules or guidelines for each chapter of this book as they pertain to student education, each student's clinical experience needs to be individualized. For example, perhaps a student is struggling on the assigned unit. The student may have made a medication error or missed an important patient assessment. Under these circumstances, it is necessary to carefully consider the appropriateness of giving the student an alternative assignment. You may not be able to observe this student at that assignment, and the student may need more time to meet the clinical objectives of the course. If this is true, do not send this student to the alternative assignment. Inform the student why this is occurring. Explain that you need more intensive time to observe his or her performance and that he or she needs more opportunity to master the objectives of this specific clinical site. Informing the course coordinator is again a wise step in case the student complains about this change.

It is also imperative that instructors document the "why" and "how" of these decisions. Many nursing programs have policies on conference forms and when or how to use them. Refer to your course coordinators for details of their expectations for documenting the performance of a student who is at risk of failing.

Essential Facts

- Alternative assignments serve many practical purposes.
- These assignments must be meaningful and approved.
- Specific clinical objectives must be established for each alternative assignment, with written and oral feedback from the student.

17

Unsafe Practice

Standards of care for nursing professionals emphasize safe and competent practice. As a result, most programs have clearly defined policies regarding safe and unsafe practice. There is zero tolerance for any unsafe practice.

In this chapter, you will learn:

- A detailed example of an unsafe practice event
- The requirements for the instructor who encounters a similar event

SAFE PRACTICE

Nursing programs have a moral and ethical responsibility to prepare graduates who will be competent and safe caregivers. Providing safe patient care is the hallmark doctrine of health care professional organizations. This obligation is clearly spelled out by the American Nurses Association (ANA). In some nursing programs, safe practice is documented as adequate knowledge of the nursing process and safe performance of skills, such as patient assessment and medication administration. In other programs, safe practice involves behaviors that uphold the ANA *Code of Ethics* (ANA, 2015). All nurses and student nurses are responsible for providing safe patient care. However, clinical educators must be aware that the concept of "safe or unsafe practice" is not commonly defined by all nursing programs.

The clinical instructor is encouraged to seek this definition in the handbook for student nurses or seek the course coordinator for assistance.

ANA's Code of Ethics

The ANA's *Code of Ethics* (2015) requires that "the nurse acts to safeguard the client and public when healthcare and safety are affected by the incompetent, unethical, or illegal practice of any person." Both students and faculty have this ethical duty. Clinical instructors have the obligation to uphold this as nurses and as faculty members. Students should be well aware of the rules and standards before beginning each rotation, which is why in most nursing programs, during the first class day of that nursing course, the student handbook is discussed in detail. Policies and elements of safe practice are discussed. Expectations of what students can and cannot do are identified and highlighted. Most schools now have student agreement forms where students, upon initial program entry, sign that they have read the student handbook and are fully aware of the policies identified.

What Is an Unsafe Event?

Exhibit 17.1 is an example of an unsafe event involving student Mary Pat and a clinical instructor. For some, it may be surprising that this is classified as an unsafe event, because it did not cause direct "harm" or may not be specifically classified as a "medication error." However, in this example, the student not only acted beyond her authorized role, but she also did not follow the nursing process by completing a patient assessment before any intervention. The clinical instructor met with the student the next day and had the student read the written report of the day's event. The student understood she was being cited for unsafe practice and that she had not properly followed the nursing process. The student confirmed her understanding by signing the bottom of the event report sheet.

ASSESSING SAFE PRACTICE

Because the *primary goal of nursing education is to train safe and competent nurses* who are accountable for their actions, clinical educators have a legal, ethical, and professional responsibility to assess students for safe practice (Smith, McKoy, & Richardson, 2001). In some cases, clinical educators may be reluctant to enforce this unsafe practice

Exhibit 17.1

Unsafe Practice Event

The clinical instructor, Cindy, was at the opposite end of the hall when she saw her student, Mary Pat, looking quite stressed. The clinical instructor quickly made her way into the room of Mary Pat's patient. She observed Mary Pat's apprehensiveness and the fact that the patient's intravenous (IV) bag was empty. Mary Pat's patient had been bathed and was reading the paper on a chair next to her bed. Everything looked neatly organized, but there was a ringing noise coming from the IV pump. It seemed that the IV bag and IV line were empty. Cindy quickly turned off the IV pump, while also clamping the IV bag. Cindy also observed that the IV tubing was looped incorrectly into the IV pump, because a key filter was not attached. She asked Mary Pat how long the IV had been ringing, and Mary Pat answered, "only a few minutes." Mary Pat shared that the patient asked to be bathed and then helped into the chair. Cindy informed Mary Pat that the pump was ringing because the bag and tubing had air in them. She also added, "Did someone come in and disconnect the tubing from the pump?" Mary Pat acknowledged that she had to disconnect the bag and tubing so that she could change the gown after the bath. Cindy picked up the nurse's assessment flow sheet and asked Mary Pat to join her in the hallway. Once in the hallway she guided Mary Pat into the clean utility room, "Do you know what was running in the IV bag?" Mary Pat looked hesitant and did not quickly offer an answer but started looking for her handwritten notes from that morning's report. She answered, "Normal saline with potassium?" Cindy commented to Mary Pat, "That bag has been infusing with heparin, which you did not document on the morning report. Two weeks ago, you also had a patient with a heparin infusion. We assessed and documented that case together. More important, the tubing was not attached to the pump correctly, so this patient may have received more heparin than she should have. Do you understand that this is a major event? We will have to report this to the primary nurse and the physician. We will also have to fill out an event report and follow the policy accordingly. But, first, let us find the primary nurse to see what he wants us to do next."

That afternoon, after the postconference, Cindy told Mary Pat to meet her in her office the next day to discuss the seriousness of the morning's event. She told Mary Pat that she saw the event as an "unsafe practice" and would need to share a written report of the situation and follow the policy on unsafe practice as documented in the student handbook. She asked Mary Pat if she had any questions regarding her comments. Mary Pat said "No," but then she quickly added, "I had taken the IV lines off the pump before . . . when I worked as a patient care technician. I sometimes had to get patients ready for their tests so I detached them from the pumps. The staff nurses have seen me do this many times."

The instructor explained to Mary Pat that even though she had worked with IVs as a patient care technician, she was functioning now only as a student—and not as a technician. Therefore, she was not allowed to disconnect IV lines during her clinical rotation without the supervision of the clinical instructor. The clinical

(continued)

Exhibit 17.1

Unsafe Practice Event (*continued*)

instructor also stressed that the role of the student was discussed extensively on orientation day and she also showed Mary Pat that it was explicitly stated in writing in the clinical handouts the students received.

The clinical instructor then followed the policy at this particular nursing program by discussing the incident with the level or course coordinator. At faculty meetings, unsafe practice events are discussed. This raises faculty awareness and draws attention to students who have "patterns" of unsafe practice events in their records. All instructors should have a thorough understanding of the nursing program's policy on unsafe practice (if any). There should not be any ambiguity in the clinical setting regarding the clinical instructor's role in the event of such situations.

---

policy because of unclear direction by their nursing programs. They simply may not have had previous experience in enforcing this policy, or they may not be sure that their student evaluation will be upheld and supported by program officials.

Failing a Student for Unsafe Practice

In addition, instructors may face challenges from failing students. Students will usually challenge upsetting academic decisions in a process that some colleges and universities call "grievance." The student's family may also become involved. All of these psychosocial aspects are challenging to the clinical instructor. It is generally more work and aggravation to fail a clinical student than to simply let the student pass. However, the ethical and legal responsibilities remain. Clinical educators are hired to assess and assist their students. Nursing programs are designed to produce students who can satisfactorily and safely perform skills.

Examples of Unsafe Practice

Instructors should be alerted to examples of unsafe practice events. There may be identified examples in student handbooks, or you may want to see the list identified by the Robert Morris University School of Nursing and Health Sciences at their website (http://snhs.rmu.edu/ForStudents/CurrentStudents/NursingPolicies/Undergraduate/UnsafeClinicalPractice).

Additional unsafe events include:

1. *The student has not prepared for assigned tasks.* The student was given an assignment to review all aspects of patient medications before administering them, but arrives on the clinical day without having looked up or prepared any of the medications.
2. *A student has not reported abnormal vital signs to the staff nurse or clinical instructor.* An adult patient had a temperature of 102°F in a postprocedure setting, but the student did not report this abnormal vital sign value.
3. *A student has given medications without the presence of the clinical instructor.* This expectation regarding medication administration is usually identified in the course syllabus and may be verbalized to students over and over again, but the event still happens. During the course of a clinical day, students will be forgetful and when provided the opportunity to give medications (pulled from the Pyxis and given to them by a staff registered nurse), they will forget and give the medications without alerting the clinical instructor. This information is in the rules and guidelines they received on their orientation day. Not following these rules should mandate an unsafe practice report and meeting.

Essential Facts

- The clinical instructor must be aware of the ANA's *Code of Ethics*.
- Each nursing program has its own definition of safe and unsafe practices, which are commensurate with state laws.

References

American Nurses Association (ANA). (2015). *Code of ethics for nurses with interpretive statements*. Silver Spring, MD: Nursesbooks.org. Retrieved from http://www.nursingworld.org/MainMenuCategories/EthicsStandards/CodeofEthicsforNurses/Code-of-Ethics-For-Nurses.html

Smith, M. H., McKoy, Y. D., & Richardson, J. (2001). Legal issues related to dismissing students for clinical deficiencies. *Nurse Educator, 26*(1), 33–38.

VI

Satisfaction in the Role

18

What Your Students Will Expect of You

Now that you are prepared to enter the world of a clinical nursing instructor, it will be important to focus on what your students will expect of you. You have clearly informed them, on their orientation day, about all of your expectations as well as those of the nursing school. Now it is time to think about their expectations of you.

In this chapter, you will learn:

- The three important attributes that students expect in a clinical nursing instructor
- What students say they expect from clinical instructors

STUDENT EXPECTATIONS OF INSTRUCTORS

You have prepared well for your new role as a clinical nursing instructor. You have read this book and used its "blueprints" to prepare for your orientation day, student evaluations, and unit orientation.

You know what you expect of yourself, but what do your students expect of you? Although they may never verbalize their expectations, students require several vital qualities in their instructor. That is why successful clinical nursing instructors remember to bring the CAP to clinical each day. This CAP is not the iconic headpiece worn by nurses in the past, but rather a mnemonic that captures the essential traits you must always exhibit to your charges:

C consistency
A approachability
P proficiency

CONSISTENCY

Nursing students are usually quite anxious on their first clinical day of each rotation. There often are rumors that upper classmates have circulated about the clinical instructor, the unit, and the workload of each rotation. The first day is often marked by shaking legs, nervous stares, and sweaty palms. This is not all bad. It is important for each student to appreciate the seriousness of the responsibility that he or she has at the clinical site, as well as the corresponding burden of responsibility borne by the clinical nursing instructor. In each circumstance, a facility's professional staff is allowing you and your students to enter their domain and care for their patients. The trust that the patients place in the facility is temporarily transferred to you.

The students must realize this and must trust you to help them navigate this unfamiliar territory. They trust you to provide adequate orientation, to establish safe limits and boundaries in terms of their roles, to ask them questions that pinpoint their areas of weakness, and to have a cohesive working relationship with the unit staff that will aid and benefit their education. Students must also be secure in their knowledge of who you are and what you expect. As such, you must exhibit consistency in your day-to-day oversight of their activities.

What does this mean? It means that you have to stick to your word and to what you have documented in handouts provided to students during orientation day or some time at the beginning of the rotation. If you say that you will e-mail their assignments to them by 4 p.m., you must do so. It means that if you say that one journal is due each week and provide the guidelines for it, you stick to that expectation and format. You cannot change the expectations after the rotation begins. Consider the examples in Exhibit 18.1.

Case Evaluation

In the Case 1, the instructor lowered her stated expectations, whereas in the second case, the instructor increased what he originally asked of his students. Both instructors lacked consistency and were ultimately

Exhibit 18.1

Consistency

Case 1
Kate is an instructor with one or two students who complain that the workload of a weekly journal assignment is too much with all of their other course responsibilities. They request that she reduce this assignment. However, most of the other students are having no difficulty completing the task and find the assignment helpful for their learning. Kate changes the assignment to resolve the complaint.

Case 2
Jerry is an instructor who tells his students on orientation day that he requires that they know the category, dose, and side effects of all of their medications. Then, on medication day, he goes further and asks them about the chemical composition, actions, and half-life of the medications.

---

unfair to their students. Vacillating expectations only serve to undermine student trust in the instructor.

Trustworthiness

Trustworthiness and consistency are intertwined. To be reliable as a nursing clinical instructor, students should often be able to predict your actions and reactions. For example, if they do not submit their journal to you on the appropriate day, they need to know from the outset that you will subtract 5 points from their grade unless they experienced a real emergency. Everyone, including the star student who is the nursing clinical genius and the struggling student who may be in jeopardy of failure, must know the policy. Consistency demands the same treatment for the same quality of work. *There can be no favoritism.*

Therefore, if you expect the students to be on the unit for clinical at 6:45 a.m., then you too are on the unit at that time. Although no clinical instructor is immune to the risk of a flat tire, a roadblock, a storm, or other situation that can delay arrival at the clinical site, these situations should be the exceedingly rare exception. Be where you are supposed to be, and on time!

Evaluation Policies

You also need to be consistent with your evaluation policies. If you say that the end of the clinical day is at 2 p.m., for example, students may ask to leave early because they have a doctor's appointment or an interview for a professional nursing job. Do not make an exception for a student unless he or she previously discussed the need for an early departure and you preapproved it. Keep in mind, however, that clinical time is valuable and already limited, so you do not want to take time away from the experience. In addition, if other students see that you are inclined to grant exceptions, you can expect them to present you with other types of early-dismissal requests.

Consistency also means if you tell a student you will supervise his or her insertion of a urinary catheter in a patient's room in 15 minutes, you are in fact there to supervise the student at the appointed time. If an emergency delays you, send a second student down to inform the first student as to why you are not there and make other arrangements. A student will become extremely frustrated if he or she is waiting for you to arrive and you do not show. The patient loses trust in the student, and the student will lose trust in you.

The trust your students place in you will be earned by the fairness and reliability that you consistently project.

APPROACHABILITY

Because students are highly anxious as they embark on a new clinical rotation, you must establish standards, guidelines, and rules. At the same time, however, you must remain approachable. What does this mean? Approachable means that you explain your rationale for your actions and ask for student feedback.

Approachable also means that you get to know each student's name and use his or her name and pronounce it correctly. Approachable means that you announce on the very first day that you understand that each student is an individual with different learning needs and different experiences. For example, some of your students may have worked as unlicensed assistive personnel or nursing technicians in health care facilities and have, therefore, learned many skills. Others may have been care providers in a different kind of facility. You must emphasize that you realize the differences and that all the objectives can be met by each student despite their varying degrees of exposure to working in a health care setting. State emphatically that you want students to tell you when they do not know something. The benefits of this policy are shown in Exhibit 18.2.

Exhibit 18.2

Approachability

During her psychiatric rotation, a senior student was responsible for taking the blood pressure of the patients on the unit. She seemed very upset by this assignment and explained to the instructor that on her job, she took blood pressure using a noninvasive automatic blood pressure cuff and had therefore forgotten how to take blood pressure manually. It was important for this senior nursing student to feel that the instructor was approachable in this situation. It allowed the instructor to review the student's technique and required the student to return to the nursing skills lab for practice.

Fairness

It is vital for students to feel that you are approachable as they deliver care to their patients. If the student makes an error or even thinks that he or she has made an error, the student will be concerned and anxious. At the same time, the student should feel that his or her concern and anxiety are not barriers to immediately coming to you with the problem.

Being approachable does not mean that you are a buddy or friend to your students. It means that they are aware that you are there to help them succeed. Your approachability will be demonstrated by your ability to remain reasonable and emotionally controlled when your assistance is needed concurrently in multiple places, when you are behind in your schedule, or when you are just not feeling up to par. Remaining approachable is paramount for the safety of the patients and the security of the students caring for them.

PROFICIENCY

As the instructor, you are the acknowledged expert. Your students watch your technique carefully and rely on your advice. The nursing staff depends on your expertise to ensure that no harm comes to their patients as a result of student inexperience. So what exactly is your level of expertise in a field whose breadth of information and practice seemingly evolves by the day? Unless you make a continued effort to keep your knowledge current, you cannot discharge your role effectively. See Exhibit 18.3 for an example of the importance of proficiency.

Exhibit 18.3

Proficiency

At the start of the fall semester, Rhonda brought her new class to the medical–surgical floor on which she had not worked for the past 4 years. The first day quickly turned into a nightmare, as Rhonda realized that the process of dispensing medications had become automated with optically scanned bar codes. Because of the security embedded in the new technology, she had no means of accessing the system and no idea how to use it once it was accessed. The students were not able to complete the fundamental chore of administering medications, and Rhonda's credibility suffered in the eyes of staff and students alike.

Case Evaluation

How can such an unfortunate situation be avoided? Start by subscribing to professional publications. These timely periodicals can offer valuable information on how research and technical innovation are affecting nursing care, often before these innovations are widely introduced into practice. It is also a good idea to keep in touch with the nurse manager, who can be a considerable asset in this regard. Innovations are usually introduced with sufficient lead time to allow for their incorporation into the daily routine. Just as the staff nurses get on-site training, so too should you. Because it may not be appropriate or feasible to participate in the training provided to the nursing staff, take the initiative to shadow a staff nurse for the day (with permission of course). This investment of time will pay dividends later, when all student eyes turn to you for instruction in a new skill.

WHAT THE STUDENTS SAY . . .

A recently graduated RN lent this perspective as a student in a RN-to-BSN program:

Being a recent nursing school graduate, the experience of different leadership styles and impact on the group is still pretty fresh in my memory banks. While I experienced several clinical instructors during my level 2 rotations, two in particular stand out in terms of being polar opposites.

The first of the two rotations was taught by an instructor who was relatively new to the program, and whether or not that has any relevance, she proved to be the more challenging of the two. She was ... more of an autocratic leader in that she was hypercritical of the group as a whole, aloof toward individuals based on personality conflict, and as a result, the group was in a relatively constant state of duress during the rotation. Also of note, when the instructor was not present, the students would essentially "put their feet up" in what seemed to me a means of escape from the tension she exuded. The result was often late med-passes, disappearing acts by the students, and further frustration by the instructor.

In my second rotation, the instructor was just the opposite. A 30-year veteran of the nursing program, her leadership style leaned more toward participatory and democratic. Before we hit the floor, she would lay down specific goals for the group and specific individuals as needed. She would then plant herself at the nursing station and wait for us to come to her. "You're not children," she would say. "I'm here if you need help, explanation, or are presented with a task you've never done." The expectation was we would work with autonomy and maintain safety by coming to her if we were uncertain. She passed no judgment regarding anything we asked, and she was always patient when teaching us new skills. This clinical group had better time management and a more complete understanding of the patients as a whole ... it was a more cohesive experience and certainly more enjoyable!

The following summary was gleaned from an informal survey of senior students who were to graduate 1 month after this informal survey was taken.

What are the most important things that a clinical nursing instructor can share with you and teach you?

- The best clinical instructors relate to students as learners. One way an instructor can do this is by sharing a difficult situation he or she experienced as a student nurse or new nurse.
- He or she can teach us how to handle tasks and assessments without expecting us to be experts, or knowledgeable just because we read the textbook. Most people learn by doing—not reading. Teach us to perform tasks as nurses—not textbook procedures because nothing is ever textbook at clinical.
- The most important thing he or she can do is take the time to answer questions and demonstrate/discuss the main objectives for the day.

What is the best way for your clinical instructor to give feedback to you?

- If it is positive feedback, it should be given to us in the clinical setting. This helps us be more confident in our clinical work. If it is negative feedback, it should be given in a site off the clinical floor so we can work on the skill/attitude outside the clinical site and we are not discouraged in the clinical setting.
- We should receive weekly feedback in the competency evaluation instrument (CEI) or some other forms such as e-mail.
- We should receive feedback through verbal communication or on the CEI. A lot of professors care more about the specific objectives on the CEI than how students perform in clinical rotation with the patients.

What is the best way to help you for your clinical orientation day?

- Conduct the simulation lab before starting the clinical rotation. Send the schedule and syllabus before orientation day so we are prepared.
- Set clear expectations for CEI, unit schedule, and tasks to be done on a daily basis.
- Hold the skills lab prior to starting the clinical rotation rather than having it after we begin. Going through expectations on Day 1 is extremely beneficial.

What do you want from the clinical instructor on your first day of taking care of the patient?

- The instructor should give an orientation to the floor, and maybe we could meet a patient or nurse manager. We could discuss a patient's plan of care and what the nurse's duty is while taking care of that patient.
- It would be good to have the unit's routine, the pass codes for everything, CEI expectations, and a good sense of what I need to get done that day. Every instructor has different expectations, and I don't want to find out that I have been doing things wrong for the first time at the mid-term evaluation.
- Students don't want what I experienced! On my first day of my first clinical I inserted a Foley catheter and our professor said that asking questions showed we were unprepared. We should

never feel that we cannot ask questions because that makes us more nervous and leads to more errors.

What do you want to know about your clinical instructor?

- It is always good to hear about a clinical instructor's most difficult patients. It shows that no matter how much experience an RN may have, nursing is still hard and RNs are still learning every day.
- We would like to know what kind of grader the instructor is as well as his or her own clinical background.
- It would be good to know what he or she expects from us, how to obtain an "A" (that is the goal every time), and the best way to contact him or her.

Discuss your worst situation in a clinical rotation.

- In psych clinical, a patient complained to my instructor that my partner and I did not care about the patients. I was in tears. Instead of asking if I was okay, the instructor accused me right off the bat.
- My instructor made me feel so stupid at the mid-term evaluation that I almost quit the program.

Discuss your best situation in clinical rotation.

- I once had a clinical instructor who did not get mad if I did not know something. If you do not know an answer, the best instructors do not get mad. Instead of giving you the answer, they lead you to the answer by asking questions.
- My clinical instructor trusted me to perform basic nursing tasks.

What suggestions do you have for a clinical instructor?

- Remember that we are novices who have not done a lot of nursing things before. Don't penalize us for double-checking with the instructor.
- Don't ask us questions in front of patients. It makes us very uncomfortable and then if we don't know the answer, patients are hesitant to be under our care.
- Assign us to recent "grads" on units. They understand what we are going through and are relatable, friendlier, and willing to teach.

- Focus less on meeting CEI objectives and focus more on applying what we learn in class to practice. I find there is a gap there when we were just trying to meet the objectives for the day to get a good grade.

Remember that you too were once a nursing student. The expectations you had of your instructors are likely no different from those that your students now have of you. They depend on you, and they need to trust you. You will earn their trust through consistency, approachability, and proficiency. Among your students you may very well have a future nursing instructor who will emulate the example you set today.

Essential Facts

- Your students have many expectations of you.
- Anticipate student expectations and strive to meet them.
- When you enter the clinical site, do not forget your CAP: consistency, approachability, and proficiency.

19

Take Time for Self-Care

Who was it who said that one cannot care for others if they do not first care for themselves? Was it an aspiring clinical nursing instructor? I think it must have been.

You already practice self-care to some extent. When you are cold, you put on a sweater and feel immediately better. The cold has not diminished at all, but you have taken a simple step to blunt the discomfort it is causing you. That is self-care in a physical sense, but the same principle extends to your mental or emotional self.

Continually responding to the many and varied needs of students over the course of the clinical rotation becomes more manageable when the clinical instructor has attended to his or her own self-care first. This chapter contains simple tools that you can begin to implement today for your daily self-care. Sharing your own self-care regimen with your students can allow them to benefit as well when they encounter stressful situations.

In this chapter, you will learn:

- The need for clinical instructors to focus on self-care to maintain satisfaction in the role
- Simple self-care practices you can adopt, including implementing simple mindfulness practices throughout the day
- How to establish "boundaries and guidelines" that define your availability to your students

THE NEED FOR CLINICAL INSTRUCTORS TO DEVELOP A PRACTICE OF SELF-CARE

In the long run, we shape our lives and we shape ourselves. The process never ends until we die. And the choices we make are ultimately our own responsibility.

Eleanor Roosevelt

Earlier in this book, we reported that you may at times notice that your students are burdened by life circumstances, the cumulative toll of which can begin to creep into their clinical performance. Well, clinical nursing instructors are human as well and thus exposed to the same type of risk. The clinical nursing instructor role is both demanding and rewarding. The rewards are easy to accept, but the demands of the job can sometimes be daunting.

Your ability to address the demands that will come your way will depend on your resiliency as a person, and that resiliency will in large part depend on how you handle stress. Making stress manageable is a conscious effort that begins with avoiding problems before they occur. Foresight and planning on your part can often be the "ounce of prevention" that negates the need for a "pound of cure." Adopting the tips and tools conveyed in the preceding pages will hopefully allow you to avoid many of the potential pitfalls that await the clinical nursing instructor, along with the stress they would otherwise generate.

This leaves you to deal with the sources of stress that cannot be proactively eliminated. In that regard, consider a program of self-care. *Consider* is the appropriate term here, because self-care is indeed a choice. You will not find it as a requirement in any job description or statement of expectations issued by an employer. And it will be one more addition to your already expansive "to-do" list. Self-care is a personal practice that will involve discipline and some small investment of time each day. Even if you feel guilty when you take time for yourself, remember that you ignore self-care at your peril.

SIMPLE STEPS TO PROMOTE SELF-CARE

According to Susan Robison, author of *The Peak Performing Professor: A Practical Guide to Productivity and Happiness* (2013), faculty members admit to not taking good care of themselves. In her book, Ms. Robison describes how self-care activities that promote physical, mental, and emotional fitness and stamina lead to higher energy in work and personal life. Following are some self-care gems that clinical nursing instructors can put to use right away.

Nutrition

Nutrition is one of the aspects of well-being that you routinely discuss with patients while often neglecting the one patient that you are the most intimately familiar with—yourself. During a busy clinical day while supervising the care of several patients, many students, and keeping safety at the top of your list, meal breaks tend to be forfeited as a cost of doing business. This is a big mistake! Leave the unit for at least 15 to 20 minutes each day for some restorative "alone time." Lift your mind off of the merry-go-round so you can eat and catch your breath. Mindful eating can restore your brain's ability to focus more readily and also to tolerate the many anxiety-filled questions that your students often bombard you with during the day. Tell one or two students that you are leaving and that it is their job to inform the remainder of the students. Let one staff member know as well. If you try to tell all of your students that you are leaving the unit for 20 minutes to eat, it will take at least an hour to address their "last-minute questions." Yes, you may be behind in administering medications, nursing treatments that need doing, or notes to be written and checked. Indeed, there will always be one more thing on the list that separates you from the blissful break you have earned. Do not fall into that trap! The benefits of taking the time to nourish yourself, to be with your own thoughts, and to regroup are immeasurable, and they will allow you to return to your flock with renewed energy and focus.

Mindful Breathing

Use "relaxing sighs" to ratchet down the anxiety of the moment. Inhale through your nose and exhale through your mouth, making a quiet, relaxing sigh as you exhale. Take a long, slow, gentle breath that raises and lowers your abdomen as you inhale and exhale. Focus on the sound and feeling of the breath. As you inhale, you are bringing needed oxygen to your brain and triggering your parasympathetic nervous system to slow down and decrease the stress cycle. You can use cues throughout your daily routine to remind yourself to take three to six relaxing sighs (e.g., at red lights while driving, while placed on-hold on your phone, waiting for elevators). You may want to place small "remember to deep breathe" stickers (the stickers can be of anything) in places that cause you stress as a cue to breathe, such as on a computer, a medication cart, a phone, or maybe a particular coworker's forehead (joking).

Some Other Things to Try . . .

- Just before entering a patient room—take two steps and one long breath in, and take two more steps and one long breath out.
- Take a 10-minute break outdoors and focus on breathing and the sounds of outside.
- When walking down the corridor, walk slowly for a brief interval, and literally concentrate on the feel of the floor beneath your feet.
- Complete the One-Minute Breathing Space exercise for self-care (see Appendix E).

Jon Kabat-Zinn's book *Catastrophe Living*, based upon his extensive body of research, is largely responsible for the modern-day focus on the ancient value of mindfulness. In 1979, Kabat-Zinn developed the "Mindfulness-Based Stress Reduction" program, the tenets of which form the basis for this chapter as it relates to utilizing some of these tools for your self-care. He offers several additional suggestions:

- When you awake in the morning, take a few quiet moments to affirm that you are choosing to go to work or school today.
- When you are in the shower, be in the shower and try not to have your workmates, students, and the meetings for the day be in there with you. Feel the water hit each part of your body.
- After you park your car, take a moment or two and just breathe, walk in mindfully, and try a smile (or even a half smile).
- At work, take a moment from time to time and monitor your body sensations. Is there tension in the shoulders, face, hands, or back? Consciously let go of tension as best you can as you exhale and shift your posture mindfully.

Take Control of What Can Be Controlled

Create boundaries for your students. You are not on call 24/7 for your students. Many of those teaching clinical nursing do so as a part-time job, primarily because they have other obligations that they must also attend to. Establish a policy on Day 1 explaining the best way that students can reach you (call, text, e-mail), and add that you need 24 to 48 hours to respond to most nonurgent inquiries that are communicated in this fashion. Try to limit work associated with clinical during your time off. Explain early on that you will need at least 1 week to deal with all submitted paperwork and return it to students. You have many hats to wear and you need to a chance to recoup.

Limit the amount of clinical rotations and employers you serve concurrently. Although the dancing dollar signs may tempt you to add that extra clinical rotation to your already heavily booked schedule, *don't do it*. You need to maintain your reserve of energy to be safe and be satisfied.

SELF-CARE AND YOUR STUDENTS

Dedicated clinical nursing instructors are a real commodity today. You are invaluable and are urgently needed to educate the vast number of students who feel that the nursing profession is the one for them. It has never been so challenging to be a clinical instructor as it is today. The number of students entering the field with preexisting mental health disorders, much debt to pay for their education, and misguided notions of what the nursing profession is really all about has never been higher. With that in mind, you need to enter each clinical day fully ready and present to assist and teach your students, keeping patient safety at the top of your priority list. One cannot do that and remain satisfied in the job without self-care and incorporating it throughout the day. You can be the students' role model by taking the time for yourself and fostering that mind-set for all of your students. They will thank you for it—eventually.

If you try self-care tools for yourself and find them helpful, why not share them with your students? As noted in the beginning of this chapter, students arrive on your doorstep with their own personal travails. For their part, the clinical site is a scary place that no amount of classroom and simulation lab instruction can ever completely prepare them for. Moreover, in today's world of immediate gratification as demanded by cell phone calls, social media pronouncements, cyber news bulletins, and an unending barrage of text messages, it is not surprising that students' ability to maintain focus on the patient and task at hand can be tenuous. Combine their emotional fragility, performance anxiety, and fragmented focus, and you have discovered that at least some (and perhaps many) of your students would also benefit from learning about self-care measures.

Fortunately, assisting nursing students in developing their ability to destress and focus is achievable with some effort on the part of the clinical instructor. In preconferences and postconferences, something as easy as introducing a 3-minute breathing exercise, or having each student lead a very short meditation (personal choice or a YouTube selection) are bookends to the clinical day that can increase focus and reduce stress. Research supports this conclusion. Morrison, Goolsarran, Rogers, and Jha (2014) found that following a 7-week training program during an academic semester at a U.S. university, students engaging in mindfulness training showed greater sustained attention in task performance and lower self-reported mind wandering during task completion than the control students who received no training.

Students generally appreciate this attention to them as individuals, and their response tends to be very positive. Many may even teach stress reduction measures to the patients they are assigned to. Here is a sampling of student comments:

I have been incorporating more mindfulness into my routine now that I take the train to work because I find it to be the perfect time, although not the perfect environment. Again, feel free to share my experience! I hope it can help someone else.

Ryan

I swear to you your mindful meditation has been an absolute lifesaver when . . . the test got so difficult. During my NCLEX I got 25 "select all that apply" questions. I had to take a break and mentally refocus because I was getting so frustrated! The deep breaths really calmed me down though and helped me focus when I was feeling so frazzled. I used them in my interview too since I was so nervous.

Jen

I have been practicing mindfulness body scan several times a week and it is really helping to keep me focused and feeling clear and calm—so thank you once again!

Alexis

Essential Facts

- Self-care is vital to the successful clinical nursing instructor.
- Self-care practices are easy to adopt and incorporate into your daily routine.
- Nursing students can also benefit from any self-care practices you share with them.

References

Kabat-Zinn, J. (1990). *Full catastrophe living: Using the wisdom of your body and mind to face stress, pain, and illness.* New York, NY: Delacorte Press.

Morrison, A., Goolsarran, M., Rogers, S., & Jha, A. (2014). Taming a wandering attention: Short-form mindfulness training in student cohorts. *Frontiers in Human Science.* Retrieved from http://journal.frontiersin.org/article/10.3389/fnhum.2013.00897/full

Robison, S. (2013). *The peak performing professor: A practical guide to productivity and happiness.* San Francisco, CA: Jossey-Bass.

VII

Of Growing Importance

20

Letters of Reference

This chapter focuses on the growing importance that prospective employers place on letters of reference written by clinical nursing instructors. Address this topic with your students on *orientation day* to set their expectations in this regard appropriately. Before you do, consider these questions: What is your legal responsibility to provide these letters? What do nurse recruiters say about the value of reference letters? How can you write a meaningful and valuable letter in a specific time frame when you have so many other responsibilities? Sample letters of reference are provided in Appendix F.

In this chapter, you will learn:

- The importance of establishing written guidelines for your students regarding your "rules" for letters of reference
- How to navigate the scenario when a "not-so-high flier" requests you to write a reference
- About online surveys from employers and agencies such as "skillsurvey.com" and what may be expected of you in completing these surveys

AN EXPERT'S PERSPECTIVE

In the year 2016, 42,537 candidates from all types of educational programs had taken National Council Licensure Examination (NCLEX) as of October 20, according to the National Council of the State Boards of Nursing (NCSBN). Most of these new aspiring nurses had one thing in common—they needed at least one letter of reference from their nursing instructors in their pursuit of jobs.

As a clinical nursing instructor, just how valuable is your letter of reference for a particular student? Perhaps this question is best answered by the employer. Rita Linus, nurse residency coordinator/nursing student facilitator for Main Line Health System in Pennsylvania, kindly offers the following insights for all clinical nursing instructors:

What are you looking for in letters of reference?

Clear descriptors of their performance are always welcome.

It is great to see where they rank in the educator's experience estimation. If they say the job candidate is one of the best students they ever instructed or falls into the top 5% of students, this makes it pretty easy!

What have you seen in letters of references that would be a "turnoff"?

General, nondescriptive letters offer little value to a nurse recruiter.

How much weight do the letters of reference really have in the nursing job hire process?

In evaluating a nursing candidate, a letter of reference represents about 30% of the total application screening tool.

What might be a "red flag" to the employer in reviewing these letters?

Narrative form letters that just change student names and offer little or no insight as to the job applicant's performance are a red flag. Conversely, template evaluations for ranking student performance are nice because they are based on consistent criteria, and comments in addition to those measures are greatly appreciated.

Do you prefer receiving recommendations from clinical instructors or classroom instructors?

In the hiring process, letters of recommendation from clinical nursing instructors are requested.

What area of clinical instruction specialty do you find to be the most helpful?

That can vary. If they are applying for OB, it is nice to see an OB clinical recommendation. Just an aside . . . often we see recommendations from psych rotations and/or community study. These are value-added as well but if the applicant's interest is ICU, it does not provide us with as much clinical experience as a leadership rotation or tele/ICU experience.

Final words from Rita . . .
In our evaluation of their application, we look at leadership/participation, volunteer activity, and professional organization membership, as well as current and past work experience (nursing and nonnursing). Some applicants do not identify their leadership activities, which can hurt them during scoring of the application.

RISKS AND GUIDELINES

Are clinical nursing instructors "legally bound" to write letters of reference? For the most part, the answer is no. Morally and ethically, though, you need to be willing to write meaningful and relevant reference letters for today's students to help them procure a job. A GPA of 3.99 may look good on a résumé, but employers want to know more. How do they function in the real world of acute nursing? How do the patients respond to them as students and caregivers? How do they get along with their peers? Do they exhibit leadership skills on the clinical unit? These strengths (or perhaps weaknesses) cannot be garnered from a GPA.

Nursing is such a unique profession utilizing cognitive and interactional skills that employers are now looking for the total package. Most prospective employers invite each candidate in for an interview where the candidate may face up to six interviewers. Another institution may do group interviews, where each candidate is asked to answer questions in a group setting.

Guidelines to decide if you are in a position to write a letter of reference for a former student would be to pose the following questions to yourself before agreeing to write a letter:

- Do you really know the student well enough to describe his or her abilities in a positive and convincing manner?
- Can you be forthright in your letter and deliver an accurate and positive portrayal of the student?
- Can you meet the student's response time frame for this employer, which often is less than 1 week?

An affirmative answer to each of these questions usually means that you are an appropriate choice to write this important document.

A WORD TO THE WISE

To save yourself countless tears and "emergency" e-mails and calls, establish clear, written guidelines for your students for distribution on orientation day. A sample guideline could be:

I am available to write reference letters after you have completed your clinical rotation with me. I need a minimum of 2 weeks notice, a written request from you stating to whom the letter should be addressed, what position you are applying for, and your signature giving me permission to write the reference letter. (Note: An e-mail request is an appropriate alternative.)

Most employers want to see school letterhead on all letters of reference and many prefer a paper letter.

Today, many schools have career counseling centers where students create an online file folder that will contain their letters of reference and other pertinent academic information relating to their job pursuit. For you, the process begins with your receipt of a student request (most often an e-mail similar to the one found in Exhibit 20.1) asking for your recommendation as the clinical instructor. You compose the letter of recommendation and submit it online with an electronic signature. Thus, the students have a permanent electronic file that can be used for years to come and they need not contact you again unless the employer requires more information.

Exhibit 20.1

Student Request for a Letter of Recommendation

Dear Professor,

I hope you are well and enjoying your summer! I took a week off after completing the Review course to relax and rejuvenate. I am now beginning my job search.

I am applying to Calmness Medical Center and have begun the process, which requires a brief survey to be completed by clinical instructors about the quality of my work as a student. Would you complete this brief reference survey? It will be sent to you via e-mail from a company called Checkster that facilitates the reference check process. You will receive the link to the survey this week.

Thank you in advance for your time and help.

Best wishes,
John Smith, Class of 20XX

Exhibit 20.2

Online Survey Sample Question

Utilizing a scale where 1 = no respect, 4 = average respect, and 7 = total respect, please indicate how you rate your respect of [Student Name] in the following areas:

1. Customer service
2. Quality focus
3. Accountability
4. Values diversity
5. Teamwork

As you can see, agreeing to write a letter of recommendation for a student is not a "once and done" type of endeavor. You need to remain available for this purpose, including your ability to truthfully answer detailed questions about the candidates long after they have left your oversight. Receiving a recommendation request more than 2 years after teaching the student in question is a possibility.

Keep in mind that your job is not necessarily done after you write a letter of recommendation. As each employer begins to seriously consider your student as a prospective employee, you may be asked to complete an online questionnaire from the hiring institution or a partnering outside vendor such as Checkster (Exhibit 20.2). This evaluation can consist of 25 or more questions and often needs to be completed within 48 hours.

Keep a file of these written requests or a folder on your computer labeled "requests for letters of reference." You may currently be on the best of terms with the student requesting the reference letter, but later on, if the student does not get the desired job, your status may change. Maybe your letter describes quite accurately a moderately successful student. If that student does not get the job, your accurate letter may be fuel for the student's anger. Having the ability to produce a signed request from the student will save you much angst in defending your role in the hiring process. Remember, too, that phone references absolutely need a signed specific release from the student.

RECOMMENDATIONS REQUESTED BY NOT-SO-HIGH FLIERS

Sally, that personable and fun student who gave you that Starbucks gift card as a token of appreciation after her clinical rotation, now asks you to write a reference letter in connection with a job application for the intensive care unit (ICU) of a very busy center-city hospital. As much as you truly enjoyed this student's company, she was not the most competent and skilled practitioner. You could see Sally doing well on a slower-paced community hospital's transitional care unit but not in the hectic environment of a metropolitan ICU. What do you do? Do you exaggerate or "stretch" the truth about Sally's abilities? Ethically, you cannot. Remember that you are being trusted by employers to give an accurate description of your students. Indirectly, but more importantly, you are being trusted by the patients your student will care for. Rather than write a letter that you do not feel comfortable with, why not change gears and engage in some career counseling? You could speak with Sally and communicate your heartfelt belief that she will make a wonderful nurse who will enjoy a long career in the right setting. Although there is no guarantee as to how your response for a letter of recommendation will be received in such an instance, there is no denying that your student will benefit the most from this honest answer.

COMPONENTS OF A GOOD LETTER OF REFERENCE

A good letter of reference will simply tell the truth. If you do not remember the student's performance, say so to the student. Give examples of the student's work when you write your letter. For example, if the student is applying to work on an oncology unit and cared for a patient with cancer during your clinical, give that experience as an example. If the student assisted all of his or her peers and the staff in an above-average manner, give that as an example. If the student rarely was on time for clinical, you may want to refer to the fact that "early morning" hours may not be the best shift for this student. It usually will be up to the student to decide to submit your letter.

It is best to state in the reference letter that you are writing at the request of (name of student) and include the capacity in which you know the student (e.g., I was the student's first medical–surgical clinical instructor in her junior year). See Appendix F for a sample letter of reference. Be sure to use nursing school letterhead.

Another tip would be to specify what job or position your reference is intended to cover. For example, if writing a letter for a new graduate, state that this student would be a qualified and excellent candidate for a new graduate position at your facility. That will prevent your letter from being misconstrued as a blanket recommendation that would include a more advanced position for a new graduate.

Ideally, you will be writing the letter to a specific person for a specific job. However, that ideal is not always the best fit in meeting student needs. Sometimes, students request a more general reference letter when they are applying to multiple facilities at multiple locations. In this situation, be accurate and specify that the letter is written for a new nurse graduate and simply describe your experience with him or her.

Today, many students requesting reference letters must waive their right to read the reference from you. Still, be cautious about what you write and only write exactly what you can support. One never knows what path this letter may take and who may ultimately read it! When no such waiver exists, it is best practice to give the student a copy of your letter before you send it to the employer. That way, if the student does not like what you have written, he or she can choose not to include your reference.

HOW TO POLITELY SAY "NO"

Nursing schools view providing recommendations on behalf of students as part of the clinical nursing instructor's job. However, this does not mean that you are obligated to provide a recommendation for a student who, in your opinion, does not deserve one. Suppose a student requests that you write a letter of reference for a job. Unfortunately, this student barely passed your clinical course. So, how can you write a letter of reference on this student's behalf? Are you required to do so? Unless a given nursing school's policy in this regard says otherwise, the answer is *no*—you are not required to write a letter of reference for any student. To avoid hurt feelings, try a subtle escape. You might say to the student that you do not feel that you are the best person to write the letter of reference, and that a different instructor with whom the student has had a more positive experience may be a better choice. If the student insists that the letter should come from you, you can write one that simply describes the clinical that you taught, that the student "arrived every day and was on time" if in fact that was the case. When that is the extent of your letter, the nurse recruiter will be able to ascertain your unwritten sentiments and, hopefully, the student will too.

GET THAT LETTER INTO THE MAIL

Pay attention to submission timeline requirements. Even a sparkling letter of reference can lose its luster if submitted late. At the same time, tardy reference requests on the part of students and your own conflicting professional priorities can sometimes make late submissions inevitable. In cases where you are simply too swamped to get a letter of reference out on time, follow up as soon as possible and apologetically explain your plight to place the "blame" where it belongs.

Considering the importance that letters of reference play in nursing job prospects, give serious consideration to these requests as you receive them, and do your best to provide an accurate and timely portrayal of your students in any letter that you do choose to write.

Essential Facts

- Establish guidelines for reference letters on your orientation day with student groups.
- In composing letters of reference, state the truth and give specifics when possible.
- Politely say "no" to a reference letter request with which you are not comfortable.

21

Role of Simulation

Clinical learning using simulation has risen in popularity. Simulation has been integrated in almost every nursing course. This chapter explores the current use of simulation and the overall role it currently plays in many nursing programs.

In this chapter, you will learn:

- The utility of simulation as an instructional method
- That simulation technology has become part of nursing curricula
- The basic application of simulation in clinical education

BACKGROUND

Simulators and simulation-type experiences are not a new phenomenon to many professionals. Simulations have been present in society for some time, as the airline industry and the military have used simulated environments to prepare their pilots or their military personnel for certain real-life scenarios (Hayden, 2010). In addition, the methods integrated in the "simulated" learning experience, such as role play, have been around since the advent of pedagogy and higher education methods. Role play has long been used by nurse educators as a teaching strategy, in which students take on roles and practice these roles based on various patient cases, or by further developing a scenario that may have occurred during that week's clinical practice experience. However, with enhanced technology, role-playing in nursing education has expanded to incorporate a lab setting with manikins and various other equipment. This type of learning has been integrated in many nursing programs as part of the "simulation" experience. To create more realism in these simulated experiences, various acute-to-more complex patient scenarios have been incorporated, as well as key practice aspects that you may find in many hospital settings. Hospitals alike have incorporated simulations to reinforce knowledge, advance skills, and evaluate the decision making of their staff personnel.

SIMULATION IN NURSING EDUCATION

In the past, simulators were primarily limited to a rubber body or body part such as a model patient or arm. This then expanded into more popular use by various nurse educators, who found themselves needing newer ways to teach challenging critical care concepts and to explore real-life patient cases without the stresses invoked by hospital settings. Simulation labs became commonplace for teaching students critical care concepts (Morton, 1995). Today, the use of simulation in nursing education has greatly expanded. The type of simulation that is selected by the educator depends on the degree of realism (or fidelity) encountered in the event. High-fidelity simulation is the type that has emerged in popularity in nursing programs since the 1990s (Goldsworthy & Graham, 2012), although there are also low- and medium-fidelity simulations. High-fidelity simulation has increased in popularity because of the computerized manikins and the conversations that can take place between students and manikins with voice-over technology. The model arms of yesterday are being replaced with this state-of-the-art equipment.

Simulation in nursing education provides opportunities for students to think and care for diverse patients in a nonthreatening, safe, and controlled environment (Jeffries, 2005). It can be seen as an instructional method that supplements learning outside of the usual classroom lecture, or as an instructional method that can highlight particularly difficult subject matter such as end-of-life care, care of the acutely ill patient, or culturally sensitive care. In some institutions, interprofessional partnerships centered on simulation experiences have become the norm. These interprofessional partnerships are well documented as the future of health education.

Today, the literature recognizes that nurse educators are using simulation to supplement their clinical education. Technology has played a large role in the surge of simulation labs that are now common in many prelicensure programs. In simulation labs, there are human patient simulators that can talk, emit various breath or cardiac sounds, and perform various other functions. These human patient high-fidelity simulators are attached to cardiac monitors and are operated through computer programs managed by simulation personnel.

Although simulation has been welcomed by many nurse educators, there are still challenges faced by nursing programs that wish to use various types of simulation experiences. Budget and personnel are key factors. There must be adequate resources and well-equipped simulation labs. Whether low- or high-fidelity simulations are used, someone must be savvy with the various computer-generated programs that are required to run a successful simulation. This person will be employed by the school and may be seen as a "simulation coordinator" with dedicated simulation personnel. This team must give attention to detail when maintaining the equipment. Last, they must have the management and communication skills to work with a variety of nursing faculty and students. Certain clinical instructors may be employed in nursing programs where there is a built-in "skills lab" prior to beginning the clinical practicum; it may be the duty of that instructor to visit and orient himself or herself to the simulation lab and to meet any assigned simulation personnel.

The prevalence of simulation and its utility in learning environments has been well documented, but questions remain regarding the role and outcome of simulation (Hayden, 2010; Norman, 2012). Initial simulation experiences were brought on by barriers found in clinical education. There continue to be restrictions imposed by agencies because of the lack of clinical sites that can accommodate students from various nursing programs. Faced with increased enrollment, the faculty shortage, and agency restrictions, clinical simulations are being seen as a teaching and learning strategy. Many are excited about its implications for clinical education and student outcomes.

LANDMARK STUDY PROVIDES EVIDENCE

The National Council of State Boards of Nursing (NCSBN) commissioned a landmark study that explored critical questions pertaining to simulations. Five associate degree programs and five baccalaureate degree programs were chosen to participate in this national study exploring the role of simulation in prelicensure nursing education. The NCSBN simulation study concluded that up to 50% of simulation can be effectively substituted for traditional clinical experiences in all core courses across the nursing curriculum without compromising learning outcomes (Hayden, Smiley, Alexander, Kardong-Edgren, & Jeffries, 2014). As a result of this landmark study, state boards of nursing are beginning to address and support simulation in clinical education. One state, Texas, has revised its education guidelines to assist their nursing schools with the use of simulation experiences. According to the Texas Board of Nursing (2015), simulation experiences in the lab can be counted as clinical experience hours (see the guidelines at www.bon.texas.gov/pdfs/education_pdfs/education_nursing_guide lines/3.8Clinical_Learning_Experiences/3-8-6-a.pdf). It further defines simulation and how it can be used for instruction.

BEST PRACTICE

Simulations are still the main responsibility of full-time teachers and not the adjunct clinical faculty. Most programs now have simulation experiences integrated into all nursing courses, from fundamentals to management courses. Clinical faculty need to be aware that today's students are now practicing assessment and fundamentals skills on a manikin in a simulation exercise during lab hours. Students who look relatively comfortable with rapidly changing aspects of their patient care may tell you that it is attributed to simulation experiences. With simulated learning, students work with high-fidelity manikins with multiple issues, to apply the nursing process to several patient case scenarios.

Simulations are here to stay. Hopefully more research can address the questions that apply to clinical education and simulation. In the future, best practices in simulation will be explored and identified in the literature. Despite all the advances with simulation experiences and simulated learning, it is imperative that all nurse educators in and out of the classroom keep an eye on their learners. The inherent job of the teacher is to know his or her learners very well and to be mindful of their "level" of learning with all types of instructional methods.

Essential Facts

- Simulation provides opportunities to practice nursing skills.
- Using simulations should be based on the level of the learner.
- Clinical instructors should be aware that most students have had simulation experiences as part of their nursing program.

References

Goldsworthy, S., & Graham, L. (2012). *Simulation simplified: A practical handbook for critical care nurse educators.* Philadelphia, PA: Lippincott Williams & Wilkins.

Hayden, J. (2010). Use of simulation in nursing education: National survey results. *Journal of Nursing Regulation, 1*(3), 52–57.

Hayden, J. K., Smiley, R. A., Alexander, M., Kardong-Edgren, S., & Jeffries, P. R. (2014). The NCSBN national simulation study: A longitudinal randomized, controlled study replacing clinical hours with simulation in prelicensure nursing education. *Journal of Nursing Regulation, 5*(2), 1–66.

Jeffries, P. (2005). A framework for designing, implementing, and evaluating simulations used as teaching strategies in nursing. *Nursing Education Perspectives, 26*(2), 96–103.

Morton, P. (1995). Creating a laboratory that simulates the critical care learning environment. *Critical Care Nurse, 16*(6), 76–81.

Norman, J. (2012). Systematic review of the literature on simulation in nursing education. *ABNF Journal, 23*(2), 24–28.

Texas Board of Nursing. (2015). *3.8.6.a. Education guideline. Simulation in prelicensure nursing education.* Retrieved from https://www.bon.texas.gov/pdfs/education_pdfs/education_nursing_guidelines/3.8Clinical_Learning_Experiences/3-8-6-a.pdf

Appendices

Appendix A
An Example of Guidelines for Clinical Orientation Day

WELCOME TO 2 SW

Orientation day begins at 8 a.m. sharp. Meet at the Barden Lobby. Directions are provided and you also can access the clinical settings website at www.lifecare.org.

September 1, 20XX
 This is a regular clinical day with time allocated for lunch. The schedule is 8 a.m. to 2 p.m.
 Bring blood pressure cuff, stethoscope, pen, paper, and notebook, and wear full uniform with identification badge per the student handbook. Expectations for students will be discussed during this orientation day.

Park in the hospital garage; you will receive parking vouchers for each day. They cannot be replaced. The fee for parking is $8.00/day without vouchers.

There will be a medication quiz on this orientation day per level policy. You must pass this quiz to begin giving medications at the site. Safe knowledge and administration of medications are evaluated at all times. You may use a calculator. For preparation help, see Blackboard under "Clinical" for examples of the medication quiz.

2 SW is an approximately 30-bed surgical unit. There are also designated beds for short stay after surgical procedures. Please review surgical procedures in your medical–surgical textbooks. You will probably have an opportunity to irrigate nasogastric tubes, change dressings, provide postoperative care, give discharge instructions, give subcutaneous insulin and Lovenox, complete assessments, perform sterile gloving for hygiene and personal care, prioritize care, review pain management, and have an observational experience requiring self-preparation in the operating room.

Please begin to review all of these procedures. You are expected to review any skill needed in the lab with the lab staff. Please make an appointment for the skills lab for the review before our first clinical day. I expect you to have reviewed all of these skills and have practiced in the lab before a clinical opportunity to perform that skill occurs.

This is a fast-paced unit, and there are registered nurses, patient care techs, aides, and a unit secretary.

Unit coordinator is Diane Marag.
Unit manager is Mary Beth Brouty.
Unit phone number on 2 SW is 610-555-36XX.

I look forward to working with you, and the staff on 2 SW is happy to be working with you.

Prof. Susan Stabler-Haas
August 30, 20XX

Appendix B
Clinical Journal: NSL/NSG 423

WRITTEN ASSIGNMENT: CLINICAL JOURNAL

Instructor: [Name]

Starting *Week 2* of this rotation: Students must submit a clinical journal on at least one of the patients they cared for during the previous week. The student must be able to *verbalize* nursing actions and rationale during the clinical day for the patients to whom he or she is assigned. Examples will be provided. Clinical journals are to be submitted weekly on Tuesdays at postconference.

WRITTEN FORMAT OF CLINICAL JOURNAL

Include your goals and objectives for the week in your clinical journal.

1. PATIENT DATA
   a. Diagnoses
   b. PMH/PSH (past medical and surgical history)
   c. Pathophysiology of diagnoses (cite)
   d. Must compare your patient's diagnosis to the textbook and cite information from the text (cite source)
2. DOCUMENT "SYSTEMS" ASSESSMENT
   a. Refer to the example previously provided

3. DIAGNOSTIC DATA—LAB WORK—NURSING IMPLICATIONS
   a. Report *potential* diagnostics pertinent to diagnoses (e.g., chest x-ray results for CHF)
   b. Report any *actual* abnormal lab work and analyze levels related to patients
4. NURSE MANAGEMENT PLAN—Document:
   a. Two priority nursing diagnoses
   b. One short-term goal (STG) per each diagnosis (patient outcome) measurable
   c. Two nursing interventions per goal
   d. Evaluate each intervention
5. PATIENT EDUCATION
   a. Identify and analyze teaching needs (actual or potential) of patients
6. MEDICATIONS (must include generic and trade names [generic names only in National Council Licensure Examination—NCLEX])

   All medications that the patient received during your shift must be listed. You must list the name of the medications, the indication for the medications (specific to your patient), lab work needed for this medication, nursing care, dosage, and antidote, if available. Lastly, you must include the nursing education required for the patient. Many NCLEX questions are chiefly concerned with the nurse's knowledge of safety-related required teaching to patients.

   Example: Enoxaparin sodium injection (Lovenox): Anticoagulant, prevention of thromboembolism phenomena following surgical procedures, prevention of such disorders when patient on bed rest

   Labs: Monitor CBC, platelet count, check for black tarry stools, hematuria, fall in blood pressure, signs of bleeding

   Nursing education: Teach patient and family how to check for signs of bleeding, gums, stool, urine. Check for bruising. Teach about over-the-counter drugs that also contain aspirin, NSAIDs, and herbal drugs that may increase bleeding.

   Dosage: SC (adults) 30 mg. Twice daily start within 24 hours of surgery

   Antidote: Protamine sulfate

   Reason this patient received medication: Patient had surgery and was immobilized, prophylactic.

7. SELF-EVALUATION AND REFLECTION
    (Minimum of two paragraphs)
    Reflect on your week: (a) Record pertinent feelings and thoughts about the nursing role. (b) Critique your performance as a student nurse. (c) Did you achieve your goals? (d) What would you do differently? Write as if you were documenting in a log or diary.
    Evaluation Method: Clinical journals will be evaluated based on the evaluative statements from the Clinical Evaluation Tool.
8. EVALUATE the patient's psychological health. Ask the two following questions: (a) Have you experienced the feeling of sadness over the past 2 weeks? (b) Have you lost interest in activities or things that you usually enjoy doing?
    Document your assessment of the patient's mental state.

Appendix C
4 C Clinical Assignment Sheet

[Name of School]

Instructor: [Name]

Note: It is highly recommended—and often a clinical site requirement—that an assignment sheet be posted in a consistent place and that you are very clear on what each student's responsibilities for the day are.

Students arrive on the unit at 7:00 a.m. and leave for postconference at 1:00 p.m.

Student	Room number/med assignment	Patient data
Claire	Day with nurse	Rose or Jan
Kristen	63 **Meds**	Student to administer all meds except IV push meds and complete all required patient care and documentation
Cara	53 54	Student to complete all nursing care for both patients, including documentation
Neil	58 **Meds**	Student to administer all meds except IV push meds and complete all required patient care and documentation

(continued)

Student	Room number/ med assignment	Patient data
Karen	OR	Required objectives and documentation sheet on Blackboard
Amy	59 **Meds**	Student to administer all meds except IV push meds and complete all patient care and documentation
Katie	69	Student to complete all patient care and documentation
Beth	79 **Meds**	Student to administer all meds except IV push meds and complete all patient care and documentation

Appendix D
Student Report Sheet

Author: Rachel E. Yoder
Villanova University
April 2016

CHANGE OF SHIFT REPORT SPECIFICS

Shift date/time	
Floor/unit/facility	
Assigned RN or staff member	
Patient initials	
Room number	
Isolation status	
Gender	
Age	
Height/weight	
Allergies/reactions	
Code status	
Fall risk?	

Special equipment needed?	
Other	

Nurse's report on current diagnosis and most recent assessment

Past medical history if discussed during shift change

Recommended or current plan of care for this shift

Patient's Current Hospitalization and Health History

Current diagnosis	
History of present illness	

Chief complaint	
Past medical history	
Past surgical history	
Social history	Tobacco? Alcohol? Drug use?

Family/genetic history		Genogram

Spirituality assessment	Stated or documented religion (if any): Request for chaplain services?

Current Medications

Name of medication	Action, indications, dosage, frequency, side effects, nursing actions, and so forth

Pertinent Lab Values and Imaging Studies

Lab values	Imaging studies
	Test date: Test performed: Result:

	Test date: Test performed: Result: Test date: Test performed: Result:

Meeting the Patient

Have you:

- *Greeted your patient and introduced yourself and your role?* Is the patient awake or asleep? Is the patient okay (remember ABCs!)?
- *Checked wrist bands* (ID with name and DOB or MRN, allergy band, fall risk band)?
- *Performed your 60-second sweep of the room to check for potential safety hazards* (items on the floor, bed rails up, bed in locked position, oxygen hook-up ready and available, wall suction working)? Also, are Ambu bag and mask of appropriate size available, pumps running correct fluids or medications at the correct rate, are tubes and line expired, are there items within the patient's reach that should not be such as needles and/or syringes, are medications left out on tables without labeling, and so forth?

Performing the Assessment

Vital Signs (time: _____)
   BP:
   Pulse (apical and/or radial):
   Resp:
   Temp (oral, axillary, or rectal):
   SpO_2:
   Pain (time of last med: _____)
      Current rating (scale used): _____
Vital Signs (time: _____)
   BP:
   Pulse (apical and/or radial):
   Resp:

Temp (oral, axillary, or rectal):
SpO$_2$:
Pain (time of last med: _____)
    Current rating (scale used): _____

Vital Signs (time: _____)
  BP:
  Pulse (apical and/or radial):
  Resp:
  Temp (oral, axillary, or rectal):
  SpO$_2$:
  Pain (time of last med: _____)
    Current rating (scale used): _____

Additional Assessment Criteria

(These prompts are not exhaustive; further assessment parameters are likely given the unit you are on.)

General Survey (Does patient appear his or her stated age? What is the patient's behavior, expression, and cognitive status? What is the patient wearing? Who is with the patient at the bedside? *Perform abuse screening during this initial exam.*):

_____
_____

Neurologic (Note LOC, PERRLA, gag reflex, verbal responses, motor responses: what deficits are present?):

_____
_____
_____

Cardiac (Note apical heart rate and rhythm; document if any extra heart sounds are heard such as a murmur and note location on chest where auscultated, and perform check on peripheral pulses and note rate, rhythm, strength, and if equal bilaterally, capillary refill. Is any edema present?):

_____
_____
_____

Intravenous or arterial lines (Are there peripheral IVs, arterial lines, or other lines? If so, note skin condition at insertion site; proximal and distal appearance of skin and limb; whether tubing is outdated; and what fluids or medications are being administered, if any):

_____
_____

Respiratory (Is the chest symmetrical? Does it rise and fall equally? Note breathing rate, rhythm, and depth; if there is work of breathing with accessory muscle involvement; auscultate lung fields and note whether clear; and note whether crackles, rhonchi, stridor, and so on are present):

_____
_____
_____

Gastrointestinal (Look at the abdomen first, then listen (auscultate all four quadrants), and then feel (palpate for masses, pain, tenderness, if guarding is present). Ask when was the patient's last meal and bowel movement (note specifics of bowel movements):

_____
_____

Genitourinary (Assess urine output and note characteristics and amount. Is there a catheter in place? Note external genitalia in both male and female patients):

_____
_____

Musculoskeletal (What is the patient's strength and range of motion? Can the patient get out of bed or chair on his or her own and ambulate on his or her own? Describe the patient's gait):

_____
_____

Skin (Inspect skin over entire body and head, noting general texture, temperature, color, any lesions, edema, redness, scaling, hair distribution and color, and so forth):

_____
_____

Psychological Assessment (Ask the patient: Have you experienced an increase in sadness within the past 2 weeks and/or have you experienced a decrease in interest in things that normally interest you within the past 2 weeks?):_____

Does the Diagnosis Make Sense?

Pathophysiology of the Problem

_____
_____
_____
_____
_____
_____

Ask: Does the clinical picture fit the diagnosis?

_____
_____
_____
_____
_____
_____

Notes

_____
_____
_____
_____
_____
_____

POSTCONFERENCE SPECIFICS (THINGS TO KNOW BEFORE YOU GO)

Your patient's age, gender, and current diagnosis/what is the patient here for?	

What is the patient's background?	
What were your assessment findings?	
What interventions did you provide?	
What was the outcome?	
Did you have to make any referrals or request assessment by other members of the interdisciplinary team?	
What are you most satisfied with regarding this encounter? What will you change or modify the next time?	

Appendix E
One-Minute Breathing Space

Have there been times when you just needed some "breathing space?" This exercise provides a way to step out of "automatic pilot" mode and into the present moment. What you are doing is creating a space to reconnect with your natural resilience and wisdom. You are simply tuning in to what is happening right now, without expectation of any particular result. If you remember nothing else, just recall the word **"STOP."**

S—Stop and take stock Checking into head/heart/body

Bring yourself into the present moment by deliberately asking: *What is my experience right now?*

Thoughts: What you are saying to yourself; images that are coming to mind
Feelings: Joy, detachment, distress, excitement, sadness, fury
Sensation: Physical sensations, tightness, holding, lightness

Acknowledge and register your experience, even if it is uncomfortable.

T—Take a breath Directing awareness to breathing

Gently direct full attention to your breathing, to each breath in and to each breath out as they follow, one after the other. Your breath can function as an anchor to bring you into the present and help you tune into a state of awareness and stillness.

O—Open and observe Expanding awareness outward

Expand the field of your awareness around and beyond your breathing, so that it includes a sense of your body as a whole, your posture and facial expression, then further outward to what is happening around you (sights, sounds, smells, and so on). As best you can, bring this expanded awareness to the next moments. . . .

P—Proceed/new possibilities Continuing without expectation

Let your attention now move into the world around you, sensing how things are *right now*. Rather than react habitually or mechanically, you can be curious and open, responding naturally. You may even be surprised by what happens next after having created this pause. . . . Check out this website (www.palousemindfulness.com).

Appendix F
Sample Letters of Reference

SAMPLE 1

September 9, 20XX

To Whom It May Concern:

I am writing this letter of recommendation at the request of Alison Z. It is a pleasure to do so. I know Alison in my capacity as nursing instructor. I taught Alison in her first nursing classroom course, in a summer elective clinical course, and more recently in her first medical–surgical clinical rotation. It is from that perspective that I write this letter.

Alison was a very conscientious and able student in her first nursing course. She provided thorough and well-detailed work and also participated in all student groups. The summer elective clinical course took place at a skilled nursing home where she cared for several totally dependent geriatric patients and provided excellent care. Most recently, I was her clinical instructor at ABC Hospital on an acute surgical floor. She was responsible for two patients on many clinical days, and she also administered their medications. She cared for a wide variety of patients and always completed all of her work, providing excellent total nursing care.

The hospital's senior staff nurses complimented Alison on her willingness to assist all of the staff and for her enthusiasm to learn and provide total care. They encouraged her to submit her résumé to become a member of their team. She also submitted excellent journals, which demonstrated a keen ability to correlate textbook knowledge with clinical performance.

Alison is extremely conscientious and well prepared in her interaction with her patients. She is astute and has an above-average ability to understand their medical and nursing needs and deliver outstanding care.

I would strongly recommend Alison for a position as a newly graduated professional nurse in your facility. If you have any questions, please contact me at 555-525-99XX or my e-mail clinical instructor@university.edu.

Sincerely,
[Instructor name], MSN, RN

SAMPLE 2

March 24, 20XX

To Whom It May Concern:

I am writing this reference letter at the request of Andrea D. It is a pleasure to do so.

I have taught Andie in both the classroom and in the clinical area. She possesses an outstanding ability to thoroughly understand complex subjects and implement this knowledge into the clinical area.

I recently had Andie in her first medical–surgical rotation at ABC Hospital. She was practicing on an acute unit and she had several extremely ill patients. She recently took an elective Critical Care Practicum with me at ABC Hospital. This course was only available to the top tier of our nursing class. It exposed the students to all aspects of critical care nursing. Andie was one of the best students in this rotation and was complimented by the nursing staff. In fact, the primary nurse, a veteran of many years, made a special effort to compliment Andie's abilities and nursing care concerning a particular critical patient.

Andie also has a unique ability to care for both the mental and physical components of her patients. It is evident in observing Andie's delivery of patient care that her years of working as an extern have contributed to her excellence.

Andie is also an excellent contributor to all discussions and to classroom interactions. She is articulate and has many leadership qualities.

I would highly recommend Andie to your hospital as a newly graduated professional nurse. If you have any questions, please e-mail me at clinical instructor@university.edu.

>Sincerely,
>[Instructor name], MSN, RN

Bibliography

Boland, D. L., & Finke, L. M. (2009). Curriculum designs. In D. M. Billings & J. A. Halstead (Eds.), *Teaching in nursing: A guide for clinical faculty* (3rd ed., Ch. 8). St. Louis, MO: Saunders Elsevier.

Dishman, L. (2015). These will be the most in-demand jobs in 2016. Retrieved from https://www.fastcompany.com/3054142/the-future-of-work

Grant, R. (2016, February 3). The U.S. is running out of nurses. *The Atlantic*. Retrieved from https://www.theatlantic.com/health/archive/2016/02/nursing-shortage/459741

Ironside, P. M., & McNelis, A. (2009). *Clinical education in prelicensure nursing programs*. New York, NY: National League for Nursing.

National Council of State Boards of Nursing. (2016). NCLEX statistics from NCSBN. Retrieved from https://www.ncsbn.org/Table_of_Pass_Rates_2016.pdf

Index

absences
   clinical day, 98
   clinical objectives and, 125–126
   oral assignments, 129
   written assignments, 129
   zero tolerance for, 20
action, on warning signs, 99–101
adjunct faculty orientation module, 18
"aha" moments, 7, 10
aides, guidance of, 7
alternative assignments, 57, 127–133
   absences, 128, 129
   appropriate, 130
   clinical setting preparation, 132
   feedback, 130, 132
   inappropriate, 130, 131
   individualizing, 133
   program objectives, 128, 129
   purposes, 130
   samples, 131
   simulation as, 128
American Nurses Association (ANA), 135
   Code of Ethics, 61, 62, 135, 136
Amorin, Frances, 14
ANA. *See* American Nurses Association
anecdotal notes, 15, 89, 92–94

approachability, student expectations of instructors, 146–147
assignment sheet, 185–186
assignments
   absences, 128, 129
   alternative. *See* alternative assignments
   clinical rotation, 130, 132
   guidelines, 122–123
   late submission of, 97
   oral, 129
   patient care, 112–114
   planning, 122
   written, 129
at-risk students. *See* not-so-high fliers
attendance policy, 20, 56

breathing, 155–156, 197–198

calculation quiz, 52
calendar, course, 18
career counseling centers, 166
case evaluation, 144–145
case studies
   patient privacy and confidentiality, 64–65
   relationship with nursing staff, 42–44

Catastrophe Living (Kabat-Zinn), 156
CEI. *See* Competency Evaluation Instrument
checklist, instructor, 22
children. *See* pediatrics
chronic personal crises. *See* personal crises
clinical competency, 4–5
clinical evaluation
  form, 17
  of instructor, by students, 86–87
  self-evaluation, 83–84, 85
  of students, by instructor, 84–86
  tool, 17–18
  triad, 83–87
clinical group, 35–37
  final stage, 36–37
  pregroup stage, 35
  transition stage, 35
  working stage, 35–36
clinical journals, 181–183
clinical objectives, 96
  absences affecting, 125–126
  example of, 96, 106
  knowledge of, 104
  tardiness affecting, 125
clinical packet, 17–18
  academic calendar, 18
  course syllabus, 18
  practicum, 17, 18, 21–22
clinical practicum, 17, 18, 21–22
clinical rotation assignments, 130, 131, 132
clinical setting
  orientation, 8
  preparation of, alternative assignments, 132
  tour of, 58–59
clinical sites, 24–33, 41. *See also* specialties
  community health, 31–32
  late arrival at, 97–98
  maternity, 26–28
  medical–surgical, 29–31
  pediatrics, 24–26
  psychiatric/mental health, 32–33

Code of Ethics (ANA), 135, 136
communication competence, 111
community health setting, 31–32
competencies, 124–125
  mathematical, 52
Competency Evaluation Instrument (CEI), 53–55
Complio, 17
computer-generated programs, 173
confidentiality
  ANA Code of Ethics, 61, 62
  case studies, 64–65
  concept, 61–62
  family members, 62–63
  HIPAA, 61, 62, 63
  overview, 61
  social media, 63–64
  visitors, 62–63
consistency, student expectations of instructors, 144–146
  case evaluation, 144–145
  evaluation policies, 145–146
  trustworthiness, 145
contact information, 56
course coordinator, 19
  clinical warning and, 100–101
course requirements, orientation and, 52, 56
course syllabus, 18
"Creating a Fair and Just Culture Within Schools of Nursing" (Barnsteiner and Disch), 29–30

daily expectations, of students, 112
dates, clinical orientation, 56
debriefing, 115
deep breathing. *See* breathing
degree programs, simulation in, 172–173
documentation, of students, 89–94
  anecdotal notes, 15, 89, 92–94
dress code, student handbook and, 20

early warning signs. *See* warning signs

electronic file, for letters of
reference, 166, 167
emotional intelligence quotient
(EQ), 44
evaluation
case, 144–145
challenges, 104
graded clinical, 103–106
of instructor, by students, 86–87
pass/fail, 105, 106
self-evaluation, 83–84, 85
of students, by instructor, 84–86
evaluation policies, consistency
with, 145–146
expectations for new clinical
instructors, 14–17

faculty handbook, 18–19
fairness, student expectations of
instructors, 147
family members, patient privacy/
confidentiality and, 62–63
feedback, alternative assignments
and, 130, 132

generic nursing students, 33–34
graded clinical evaluation, 103–106
challenges, 104
forms, 106
overview, 103
types, 104–106
unanticipated events, 104

handbooks
faculty, 18–19
student, 19–21
health care agencies, entry
requirement, 17
Health Information Technology for
Economic and Clinical Health
(HITECH) Act, 63
Health Insurance Portability and
Accountability Act (HIPAA),
61, 62, 63
hedging, 97
high fliers

characteristics of, 70–71
identifying, 70
not-so-high fliers versus, 74
reflection journals written by, 71
high-fidelity simulation, 172
HIPAA. *See* Health Insurance
Portability and Accountability
Act
HITECH. *See* Health Information
Technology for Economic and
Clinical Health Act
hospital entry requirements, 17
hours, clinical orientation, 56

identity, development of, 3–11
"aha" moments, 7, 10
clinical competency, 4–5
clinical setting orientation, 8
communication, 7
conflicts, 7
contribution to nursing
profession, 5–6
earning, maximizing, 10
friendship with students, 6
liked by students, 6–7
motivation, 10
patient details, 8–9
patient interaction, 9
simulation experiences, 11
staff nurses/aides guidance, 7
staff supervision, 9
impaired student policy, 21
individualizing student
assignments, 133
informal meeting, 96
information list, for instructors, 49
instincts, trusting, 101
instructor checklist, 22
instructors
anecdotal notes, 15
baseline knowledge, 13–14
current evidence of liability,
15–16
information list for, 49
required knowledge for, 15
student evaluation of, 86–87

interaction with nursing staff. *See* relationship with nursing staff
interactive discussion, 5
interprofessional partnerships, on simulation, 172
intuition, warning signs and, 101
isolation standards, 8

job description, 18
journals
    clinical, 57, 181–183
    student. *See* reflection journals, by students

lab specimens, 8
late arrival at clinical site, 97–98
late submission of assignments, 97
late-arriving students, 125. *See also* tardiness
letters of reference, 163–170
    components, 168–169
    electronic file, 166, 167
    expert's perspective, 163–165
    online file folder, 166
    requesting, 167–168
    risks and guidelines, 165
    sample, 199–201
    saying "NO" politely, 169
    submission timeline, 169–170
    written guidelines, 166
level coordinator, 19
    clinical warning and, 100–101
Likert-type scale, 85, 106

make-up assignments, 128
    oral, 129
    written, 129
make-up submissions, 56–57
maternity, 26–28
mathematical competency, orientation and, 52
medical–surgical nursing, 29–31
medications
    calculation quiz, 52
    patients, 8, 9

mental health nursing. *See* psychiatric/mental health nursing
mid-term evaluation, 96
Mindfulness-Based Stress Reduction program, 156
monitoring, not-so-high fliers, 76–79
motivation, students and, 10

National Council of State Boards of Nursing (NCSBN), 116–117, 173–174
    on patient privacy, 64
    on social media, 64
NCSBN. *See* National Council of State Boards of Nursing
neonates, 27
new clinical instructors, expectations for, 14–17
nothing by mouth (NPO), 8
not-so-high fliers, 70
    characteristics of, 74–76
    high fliers versus, 74
    identifying, 73–74
    monitoring, 76–79
    red flags, 74
NPO. *See* nothing by mouth
nursing program's policies
    clinical packet, 17–18
    clinical practicum, 17, 18, 21–22
    faculty handbook, 18–19
    student handbook, 16, 19–21
nutrition, 155. *See also* self-care

online file folder, 166
online questionnaire, for prospective employment, 167
oral assignments for clinical absence, 129
orientation
    clinical dates, 56
    clinical hours, 56
    clinical setting, 8

contact information, 56
course requirements, 52, 56
expectations, 56
guidelines, 48–50, 179–180
journals, 57
key components, 56–58
mathematical competency, 52
students' goals, 52
students' responsibilities, 58
things to be done prior to semester's first day, 48–50
tour, 58–59

part-time job, 156–157
pass/fail evaluation, 105, 106
patient care assignments, 112–114
patient privacy
  ANA Code of Ethics, 61, 62
  case studies, 64–65
  concept, 61–62
  family members, 62–63
  HIPAA, 61, 62, 63
  overview, 61
  social media, 63–64
  visitors, 62–63
patient safety, 28
patients
  code status of, 8–9
  details of, 8–9
  isolation standards of, 8
  medications for, 8, 9
  NPO status of, 8
  students interaction with, 9
Peak Performing Professor: A Practical Guide to Productivity and Happiness (Robison), 154–155
pediatrics, 24–26
personal crises, 99
phone references, 167. *See also* letters of reference
policies, 19–20. *See also* nursing program's policies
  attendance, 20
  dress, 20

impaired student, 21
safe/unsafe practice, 20–21
substance abuse, 21
postconferences, 115–119
  concept, 115–116
  preconferences versus, 115
  student experience sharing, 117–119
  teaching opportunities, 116–117
postpartum woman, 27
preconferences, 111–114
  concept, 111–112
  daily expectations, 112
  overview, 111
  postconferences versus, 115
  student guidance, 112–114
prelicensure nursing education, simulation in, 173
professional liability, 92
proficiency, 147–148
  case evaluation, 148
program goals, student handbook and, 19–20
psychiatric/mental health nursing, 32–33
Publication Manual of the American Psychological Association, 129

questioning, 5

red flag warnings, 74, 96–99
  chronic personal crises, 99
  hedging, 97
  late submission of assignments, 97
  tardiness, 97
reference letter. *See* letters of reference
reflection journals, by students, 71
relationship with nursing staff, 41–46
  case studies, 42–44
  effective interaction, 44–45
  EQ and, 44

relaxing sighs, 155–156. *See also* breathing; self-care
Robert Morris University School of Nursing and Health Sciences, 138
Robison, Susan, 154–155
role-playing, 5, 171–172

safe practice, 135–136
 assessing, 136–139
 policy, 20–21
satisfactory clinical grade, 105, 106. *See also* unsatisfactory clinical grade
self-care, 153–159
 nutrition, 155
 overview, 153
 practice of, developing, 154
 relaxing sighs, 155–156
 steps promoting, 154–157
 students and, 157–158
self-efficacy, 113
self-evaluation, 83–84, 85
simulation, 11, 171–175
 as alternative assignments, 128
 best practices, 174
 challenges, 173
 clinical learning using, 171
 as instructional method, 172
 interprofessional partnerships, 172
 NCSBN study, 173–174
 prelicensure education, 173
 role play, 171–172
 type of, 172
 utility in learning environments, 173
simulation coordinator, 173
simulation labs, 172, 173
social media, 63–64
specialties, 24–33
 community health, 31–32
 maternity, 26–28
 medical–surgical, 29–31
 pediatrics, 24–26
 psychiatric/mental health, 32–33

staff, nursing
 effective interaction with, 44–45
 guidance, 7
 relationship with, 41–46
 supervision, 9
strong students. *See* high fliers
student(s)
 capability assessment, 69–70
 daily expectations of, 112
 experience sharing, in postconferences, 117–119
 friendship with, 6
 generic nursing, 33–34
 goals for clinical practicum rotation, 52
 mathematical competency, 52
 motivation, 10
 patient details, 8–9
 patient interactions, 9
 preconferences, guidance of, 112–114
 presentations, in postconferences, 116–117
 responsibilities, 58
 second-career (second-degree), 34–35
 self-evaluation, 83–84, 85
 strong. *See* high fliers
 weak. *See* not-so-high fliers
student expectations, 143–152
 approachability, 146–147
 consistency, 144–146
 overview, 143–144
 proficiency, 147–148
student handbook, 16, 19–21
 attendance policy, 20
 dress code policy, 20
 impaired student policy, 21
 program goals, 19–20
 safe/unsafe practice policy, 20–21
 substance abuse policy, 21
student journals. *See* reflection journals, by students
student report sheet, 57, 187–195
student–preceptor relationship, 5
substance abuse policy, 21

supervision
  performing skills without, 98–99
  staff, 9
syllabus, course, 18

tardiness, 97
  affecting clinical objectives, 125
  pattern of, 125
  zero tolerance for, 20
teaching opportunities, in postconferences, 116–117
  limitations, 117
  student presentations, 116–117
Texas Board of Nursing, 174

unanticipated events, 104
unplanned events, 121, 124
unsafe practice
  examples of, 138–139
  failing student and, 138
  policy, 20–21

unsatisfactory clinical grade, 105, 106. *See also* satisfactory clinical grade

verbal presentation, key components of, 56–57
visitors, patient privacy/confidentiality and, 62–63
voice-over technology, 172

warning signs, 95–102
  intuition, 101
  overview, 95
  red flags, 96–99
  taking action on, 99–101
weak students. *See* not-so-high fliers
woman. *See also* maternity
  in labor, 26–27
  postpartum, 27
written assignments for clinical absence, 129

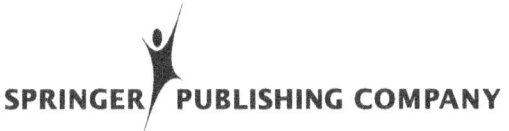

SNEAK PEEK!

Fast Facts for the Student Nurse

By Susan Stabler-Haas MSN, RN, PMHCNS-BC

Enjoy the following chapter from the perfect companion book for your students!

Written with candid humor, this Fast Facts guide features the information that nursing students really need to know in order to achieve excellence up to and beyond the NCLEX®!

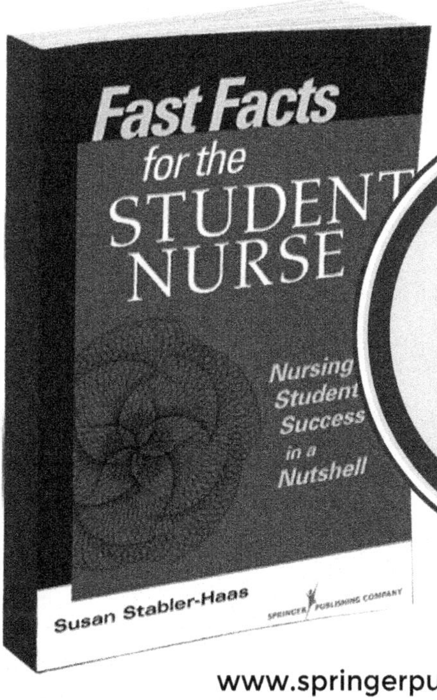

SAVE 20% Plus **FREE SHIPPING** with Code **FFPEEK**

www.springerpub.com

ESSENTIALS for the STUDENT NURSE

Nursing Student Success in a Nutshell

Susan Stabler-Haas, MSN, RN, CS, LMFT

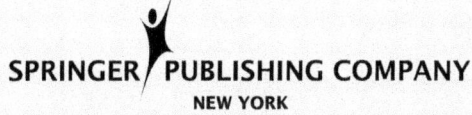

SPRINGER PUBLISHING COMPANY
NEW YORK

Contents

Foreword
Preface
Acknowledgments

Part I   YOUR NEW LIFE AS A STUDENT NURSE

1. Now That Your Journey Has Begun
2. Common Myths Regarding Nursing
3. Facing the Challenge of Your Chosen Major
   In Student Nurses' Own Words . . .

Part II   SUCCESS IN THE CLASSROOM

4. Optimizing the Value of Classroom Time
5. Interacting With Your Instructor
6. What Kind of Learner Are You?
7. The Digital World of Nursing Education
   In Student Nurses' Own Words . . .

Part III   SUCCESS AT THE CLINICAL SITE

8. The Clinical Experience
9. Once On-Site

10. Patients as People
   In Student Nurses' Own Words . . .

Part IV SUCCESS AT HOME

11. Working, Family, and Crises That Won't Wait
12. You Are Your Own Patient
    In Student Nurses' Own Words . . .

Part V SUCCESS FOLLOWING GRADUATION

13. Licensure
14. NCLEX® (The National Council License Examination)
15. The Basics of Job Hunting in Nursing
16. The Fine Points of Job Hunting in Nursing
17. Reaching for the Next Star
18. What? Me Publish?
19. Insuring Your Investment
20. A Nursing Fable
    In Student Nurses' Own Words . . .

References
Index

Preface

It had been a day like any other in the life of a seventh grader. My night had been unremarkable as well. But as I settled into bed and pulled the covers up around me, an event would occur that would one day help shape my professional life. While waiting for sleep to come, I heard the lonely and faraway cry of an ambulance. I listened as it crept closer and closer—slowly at first but then flying past my window like a Halloween ghost. I listened as its intense and mournful wail was gradually overcome by the returning stillness of the night. The ambulance had not stopped at my house, but it had managed to plant a seed in the imagination of a 12-year-old girl as it hurried by. To myself, I said, "I wonder what it would be like to be a nurse and help those who are sick."

It is curious how the most innocuous of events or the most casual of encounters can put us on a career path with no warning to ourselves and little notice by others. What made you interested in nursing as a career? Perhaps a family member or adult you admire worked as a nurse. Maybe you or someone close to you was a hospital patient, and you were intrigued by the nurses who constantly moved in and out of the room. You may have even read stories about how these wonderful and at times heroic individuals effectively combine the science of health care with the art of healing in the interest of making their patients well again. As noted in Chapter 8, *"Today's nurse is in constant motion, shuttling back and forth between the technical aspects of nursing practice and the human aspects of nursing care. There are few other professions that require their practitioners to be so adept in so many different ways. As a nurse, you can treat, educate, console, bathe, and medicate a patient all within the same day."*

Now poised to begin your life's work, you may have recently entered nursing school or are considering the possibility of becoming a nursing student. This book has been written especially for you. Its purpose is to acquaint you with the demands and rewards of both an education and a career as a nurse. Think of this book as a map of sorts that is intended to prepare you for the realities you will encounter as you embark upon your career journey. By knowing what to expect, you will be in a better position to navigate the sometimes turbulent and sometimes tranquil seas that now separate you from a nursing license.

You should first understand the perspective from which this book has been created. It is not the product of statistical research. Rather, it is a personal blend of informed observation, practical advice, and helpful hints from my experience as a staff medical-surgical nurse, a rehab nurse, an industrial nurse, a nurse manager in a critical care unit of a major urban hospital, a nurse psychotherapist, a nursing instructor in associate, diploma, and second-degree programs, a university assistant professor—and, yes, my own vivid recollections of having once been a student nurse myself. This book also represents experiences drawn from more than a thousand nursing students whom I have taught over the years. Many examples in this book are their stories, and the section at the end of each part entitled "In Student Nurses' Own Words . . . " are the real words of my former students.

I hope that this book will be your companion as you move through your nursing education program and eventually into your own nursing role. I also hope that it helps you to sustain your own mental and physical health as you progress toward your professional goal.

Finally, it is my fondest hope that you will find nursing to be both professionally and personally fulfilling, just like the girl who heard the ambulance race by her window so many years ago.

Now That Your Journey Has Begun

A career in nursing is a journey that begins with information gathering and planning on the part of the student nurse.

In this chapter, you will learn:

1. That a career in nursing requires careful preparation.
2. About the public's perception of the nursing profession.
3. About the "typical" nursing student.

A CAREER IN NURSING REQUIRES CAREFUL PREPARATION

Think back to your last vacation. Was it fun? Did you relax? Was it everything that you hoped it would be? If so, chances are that your vacation's success was the result of careful planning—where to stay, what to pack, and, most important, how to get there.

In a larger sense, the mechanics of planning a career are similar to those involved in planning a vacation. Like those glossy brochures touting the many treasures and pleasures to be found from Las Vegas to London and from Madrid to Macao, a wide array of careers has beckoned to you. After carefully considering those options, you have decided that nursing is the profession that best reflects your personal values and ambitions.

THE PUBLIC'S PERCEPTION OF THE NURSING PROFESSION

Congratulations on making a great career choice! A 2010 Gallup poll has again found nursing to be the profession most trusted by the general public. Since becoming a part of this survey in 1999, nursing has been rated the most trusted profession every year with the exception of 2001, when firefighters took the top spot. The public's trust in nurses is well placed. In addition to being caregivers, nurses are often advocates for their patients, doing what they can to help them successfully navigate the health care system. It is a trust that can be traced back to the battlefield and the contributions of nursing icons such as Florence Nightingale and Clara Barton. Chances are, however, that you were drawn to the profession by an individual who is not famous—one whose skill and dedication kindled a passion within you strong enough to illuminate your ultimate career path.

THE TYPICAL NURSING STUDENT

The typical nursing student is no longer typical. Once she was almost exclusively a young white female, but that is changing. In 1990, minority enrollment in basic registered nursing programs was 16%; this nearly doubled to 29% by 2008–2009. Similarly, male participation has doubled as well, from a level of 6% in 1988 to about 12% today. The next threshold to be crossed is age. The advent of second-degree programs to accommodate career changers interested in nursing will no doubt begin to raise the average age of the nursing student as well.

Essential Facts

- A career in nursing requires careful preparation.
- Nursing is continually rated as society's most respected profession.
- The profile of the typical nursing student is evolving to become more inclusive of males, minorities, and older program participants.

Lightning Source UK Ltd.
Milton Keynes UK
UKOW05f1527201217
314750UK00012B/558/P